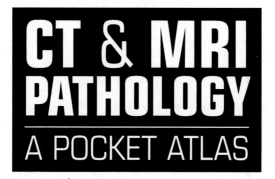

# CT & MRI
# PATHOLOGY

## A POCKET ATLAS

## Notice

Medicine is an ever-changing science. As new research and clinical experience broaden our knowledge, changes in treatment and drug therapy are required. The authors and the publisher of this work have checked with sources believed to be reliable in their efforts to provide information that is complete and generally in accord with the standards accepted at the time of publication. However, in view of the possibility of human error changes in medical sciences, neither the editors nor the publisher nor any other party who has been involved in the preparation or publication of this work warrants that the information contained herein is in every respect accurate or complete, and they disclaim all responsibility for any errors or omissions or for the results obtained from use of the information contained in this work. Readers are encouraged to confirm the information contained herein with other sources. For example and in particular, readers are advised to check the product information sheet included in the package of each drug they plan to administer to be certain that the information contained in this work is accurate and that changes have not been made in the recommended dose or in the contraindications for administration. This recommendation is of particular importance in connection with new or infrequently used drugs.

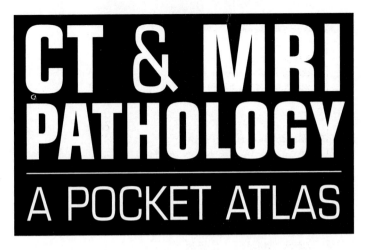

# CT & MRI PATHOLOGY

## A POCKET ATLAS

**Michael L. Grey, MS, RT(R), (MR), (CT)**

Assistant Professor
Radiologic Sciences
MRI/CT Specializations
Department of Health Care Professions
College of Applied Sciences and Arts
Southern Illinois University
Carbondale, Illinois


**Jagan M. Ailinani, MD**

Clinical Professor of Radiology and Community Medicine
Southern Illinois University School of Medicine
Senior Attending Radiologist
Memorial Hospital of Carbondale
Carbondale, Illinois

McGraw-Hill Professional

New York   Chicago   San Francisco   Lisbon
London   Madrid   Mexico City   Milan   New Delhi
San Juan   Seoul   Singapore   Sydney   Toronto

BS

**The McGraw·Hill Companies**

## CT & MRI PATHOLOGY: A POCKET ATLAS

Copyright © 2003 by The McGraw-Hill Companies, Inc. All rights reserved. Printed in the United States of America. Except as permitted under the United States Copyright Act of 1976, no part of this publication may be reproduced or distributed in any form or by any means, or stored in a data base or retrieval system, without the prior written permission of the publisher.

1234567890   DOC DOC   09876543

ISBN: 0-07-138040-X


This book was set in Times Roman by Parallelogram.
The editors were Michael Brown,  Janene Matragrano,  and Karen G. Edmonson.
The production supervisor was Richard Ruzycka.
The text designer was Marsha Cohen/Parallelogram.
The cover designer was Aimee Nordin.
The indexer was Patricia Perrier.
R.R. Donnelley & Sons was printer and binder.

This book is printed on acid-free paper.


### Library of Congress Cataloging-in-Publication Data

Grey, Michael L.
   CT & MRI pathology : a pocket atlas / Michael L. Grey, Jagan M.
     Ailinani.—1st ed.
       p.  cm.
   Includes bibliographic references.
   ISBN 0-07-138040-X [alk paper)
   1. Magnetic resonance imaging—Atlases. 2. Tomography—
Atlases. 3. Diseases—Atlases.  I. Title: CT and MRI pathology. II
Ailinani, Jagan M. Title.
   [DNLM: 1. Tomography, X-Ray Computed—methods—Atlases. 2.
Tomography, X-Ray Computed—methods—Handbooks. 3. Magnetic
Resonance Imaging—methods—Atlases. 4. Magnetic Resonance
Imaging—methods—Handbooks.  WN 17 G844c 3003]
RC78.7.N83 G747 2003
616.07'57—dc21

4/29/04

### Dedication

I would like to thank my wonderful wife Rebecca
for her support, encouragement,
and assistance in this project,
and our children, Kayla and Emily,
who were always waiting for me with open arms.
I love you.
**MLG**


To my wife Uma
and children Vasavi and Hary.
**JMA**

# PREFACE

In recent years, there has been an explosion in the technology of diagnostic imaging. The introduction of computed tomography (CT) and magnetic resonance imaging (MRI) has greatly enhanced our ability to study and diagnose disease.

This handbook provides technologists and students with CT and MRI findings of common pathologic conditions seen in day-to-day practice, along with pertinent clinical information. Each pathology listed has a single page of text accompanied with MRI and/or CT images that depict the pathology. The text includes a description, etiology, epidemiology, signs and symptoms, imaging characteristics for CT and MRI, treatment, and prognosis statements.

Obviously, many pathology textbooks are available that provide greater detail on all aspects of these conditions. This is not a textbook and is not meant to replace standard textbooks. Instead, it is meant as a source for concise review of the pathology and imaging information. Technologists can carry this handbook in their lab coat pocket and can quickly check pathologic imaging finding and clinical information when a textbook is not available.

*Michael L. Grey, MS, RT(R) (MR) (CT)*
*Jagan M. Ailinani, MD*

# ACKNOWLEDGMENTS

I am extremely thankful to my students, technologists, and the imaging facilities that have contributed to collecting and providing the images for this handbook. I would also like to acknowledge the support of my professional colleagues, especially Paul Sarvela, Steven Jensen, Rosanne Szekely, Karen Having, Don Borst, Scott Collins, and Robert Broomfield. Thanks to the leadership, advice, and patience of the editorial, production and design staff at McGraw-Hill. To Kathy, Kim, and Mary, the greatest librarians, thank you for all your assistance. Thanks to my parents Robert and Yvonne, for their support and encouragement and for teaching me diligence.

Finally, I would like to thank my Lord and Savior Jesus Christ for blessing me with the ideas that went into the design of this handbook and the energy to endure the task of seeing a dream become reality.

*MLG*

To my wife, Uma, and children, Vasavi and Hary

*JMA*

# CONTENTS

---
### PART I.
---

## Principles of Imaging in Computed Tomography and Magnetic Resonance Imaging / 1

---
### PART II.
---

## Central Nervous System / 5

BRAIN

### Neoplasm

### Congenital

### Vascular Disease

PART III.

# Head and Neck / 103

**Congenital**

**Tumor**

**Sinus**

**Trauma**

PART IV.

# Chest and Mediastinum / 123

**Lungs**

**Mediastinum**

## PART V.
## Abdomen / 143

Contents

## PART VI.
### Pelvis / 205

## PART VII.
### Musculoskeletal / 213

## Knee

## Ankle & Foot

# PART I

# Principles of
# Imaging Pathology

# Principles of Imaging in Computed Tomography and Magnetic Resonance Imaging

Since the initial discovery of x-ray by Wilhelm Conrad Roentgen on November 8, 1895, the field of radiology has experienced two major breakthroughs that have revolutionized how we look into the patient's body. The first, computed tomography (CT) came in the early 1970s. The second, magnetic resonance imaging (MRI) was initially introduced in the early 1980s.

In CT, a finely collimated x-ray beam is directed upon the patient. As the x-ray tube travels around the patient, x-rays are emitted toward the patient. As these x-rays interact with the various tissues in the patient's body, some of the x-rays are attenuated by the tissues while others are transmitted through the tissues and interact with a very sensitive electronic detector. The purpose of these detectors is to measure the amount of radiation that has been transmitted through the patient. After the amount of radiation has been measured, the detector converts the amount of radiation received into an electronic signal that is sent to a computer. The computer then performs mathematical calculations on the information received and reconstructs the desired image. This information is assigned a numerical value that represents the average density of the tissue in that respective pixel/voxel of tissue. These numerical values reflect the patient's tissue attenuation characteristics and may be referred to as Hounsfield numbers, Hounsfield units (HU), or CT numbers that range from –1000 (air) to +1000 (dense bone or tooth enamel). CT uses water as its standard value and it is assigned a Hounsfield number of 0.

To diagnose a disease process, the radiologist looks for changes in the normal density (HU) of an organ, an abnormal mass, or an altered or loss of normal anatomy. The advantages of CT include its ability to image patients that (1) have experienced trauma, (2) are suspect to having had a stroke, (3) acutely ill, (4) have a contraindication to MRI, or (5) require better bone detail that can be scanned in CT in a quick and efficient manner. In addition, since the development of helical (spiral) CT in the early 1990s with single-slice technology and further technological advances in the mid-1990s to multi-slice imaging, CT is able to perform volumetric imaging quickly and generate reformatted anatomic images in any plane (e.g. sagittal or coronal). The disadvantages of CT include (1) exposure to the radiation dosage, (2) possible reaction to the iodinated contrast agent, (3) lack of direct multiplanar imaging, and (4) loss of soft-tissue contrast when compared to MRI.

MRI incorporates the use of a strong magnetic field and smaller gradient magnetic fields in conjunction with a radiofrequency (RF) signal and RF coils specifically tuned to the Larmor frequency of the proton being imaged. An image is acquired in MRI by placing the patient into a strong magnetic field and applying a radiofrequency signal at the Larmor frequency of the hydrogen proton (42.58 MHz/T). Gradient magnetic fields are used to assist with spatial localization of the RF signal. The gradients are assigned to the tasks of slice selection, phase encoding and frequency encoding or readout gradient. In the magnet, the patient's hydrogen protons align either parallel (with) or antiparallel (against) the magnetic field. The RF signal is rapidly turned on and off. When the RF signal is turned on, the protons are flipped away from the parallel axis of the magnetic field. Once the RF is turned off, the proton begins to relax back into the parallel orientation of the magnetic field. During the relaxation time, a signal from the patient is being received by the coils and sent to the computer for image reconstruction. This process is repeated several times until the image is acquired.

There are several different types of pulse sequences used in MRI to acquire patient information. These can be grouped into proton (spin) density, T1 relaxation time, and T2 relaxation time. These pulse sequences demonstrate the anatomy differently and help differentiate between normal and abnormal structures. A combination of these pulse sequences may be used to assist with the diagnosis.

A T1-weighted pulse sequence uses a short TR (repetition time) and short TE (echo time) values to produce a high or bright signal in substances such as fat, acute hemorrhage, and slow-flowing blood. Structures such as cerebrospinal fluid and simple cysts may appear with a low or dark signal. In many cases, the pathologic process will appear with low signal in T1-weighted images.

A proton-density-weighted image uses long TR and short TE values to produce images based on the concentration of hydrogen protons in the tissue. The brighter the area, the greater the concentration of hydrogen protons. The darker the area, the fewer the number of hydrogen protons.

A T2-weighted pulse sequence uses long TR and long TE values to obtain a high signal in substances such as cerebrospinal fluid, simple cysts, edema, and tumors. Structures such as fat and muscle will appear with low signal. Many pathologic conditions present with high signal on T2-weighted pulse sequences.

MRI has several advantages such as (1) it acquires patient information without the use of ionizing radiation; (2) it produces excellent soft tissue contrast; (3) it can acquire images in the transverse (axial), sagittal, coronal, or oblique (orthogonal) planes; and (4) image quality is not affected by bone. The disadvantages primarily associated with MRI would include: (1) any contraindication that would present a detrimental effect to the patient or health care personnel; (2) long scan time when compared to CT; and (3) cost. The effects of the magnetic field, varying gradient magnetic fields, or the RF energy used pose the greatest harmful effects to biomedical implants that may be in the patient's body. Before entrance into the strong magnetic field can be obtained, everyone including patients, family members, health care professionals, and maintenance workers must be screened for any contraindications that may result in injury to themselves or others. These may include any biomedical implant or device that is electrically, magnetically or mechanically activated such as pacemakers, cochlear implants, certain types of intracranial aneurysm clips and orbital metallic foreign bodies. The contraindications focus on devices that may move or undergo a torque-effect in the magnetic field, overheat, produce of an artifact on the image, or become damaged or functionally altered. Most magnets used in MRI are superconductive and the magnetic field is always on. Any ferromagnetic material (e.g., O2 tank, wheelchairs, stretchers, scissors, etc.) may become a projectile and potentially cause an injury or death when brought into the magnetic environment.

# PART II

# Central Nervous System

# BRAIN
## NEOPLASM

## ACOUSTIC NEUROMA

**Description:** An acoustic neuroma, also known as a vestibular schwannoma is a benign fibrous tumor that arises from the Schwann cells covering the vestibule portion of the eighth cranial nerve. These tumors are well encapsulated, compress but do not invade the nerve. Acoustic neuromas account for approximately 80- to 85 percent of all cerebellopontine angle (CPA) tumors and make up 10 percent of all intracranial tumors.

**Etiology:** There is no known cause for this tumor. Bilateral 8th cranial nerve schwannomas are pathognomonic for neurofibromatosis type II.

**Epidemiology:** Acoustic neuromas account for approximately 5 to 10 percent of all intracranial tumors. They are the most common tumor affecting the cerebellopontine angle. Males and females are affected equally. The average age of onset is between 40 and 60 years.

**Signs and Symptoms:** Sensorineural hearing loss, tinnitus, and vertigo are common in patients.

**Imaging Characteristics:** Note: MRI is the imaging modality of choice.

### CT
• Well-rounded hypodense to isodense mass on non-contrast study.
• Hyperdense with contrast enhancement.

### MRI
• T1-weighted imaging without contrast is usually isointense to slightly hypointense.
• T1-weighted pulse sequence with contrast enhancement demonstrates the tumor with a marked enhancement.
• T2-weighted images may demonstrate an increase (hyperintense) in signal.
• Baseline imaging following surgery should include a precontrast T1 and fat-suppression post-contrast pulse sequences.

**Differential Diagnosis:** Includes mainly meningioma, metastasis, and paraganglioma.

**Treatment:** Surgery intervention is required.

**Prognosis:** Depending on the size of the acoustic neuroma, the prognosis is encouraging and usually is curative.

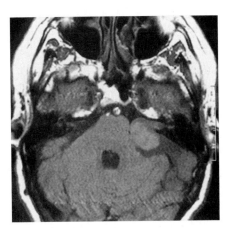

**FIGURE 1. Acoustic Neuroma.** Noncontrast T1-weighted axial image demonstrating round isointense mass at the left cerebellopontine angle.

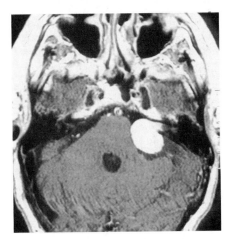

**FIGURE 2. Acoustic Neuroma.** Post-contrast T1-weighted axial image demonstrating an intense contrast enhancing extraaxial mass at the left cerebellopontine angle close to the left internal auditory canal (IAC) consistent with an acoustic neuroma.

# Brain Metastasis

**Description:** Brain metastasis is the metastatic spread of cancer from a distant site or organ to the brain.

**Etiology:** Metastatic dissemination to the brain primarily occurs through hematogenous spread.

**Epidemiology:** Metastases to the brain accounts for approximately 15 to 25 percent of all intracranial tumors. Brain metastases may involve the supratentorial or infratentorial parenchyma, meninges, or calvaria. Most metastases to the brain parenchyma develop by hematogenous spread from primary lung, breast, gastrointestinal tract, kidney and melanoma tumors. Metastases to the calvaria may result from breast and prostate cancers. Metastases to the meninges may result from bone or breast cancer.

**Signs and Symptoms:** Depending on the extent of involvement, the patient may present with seizures, signs of intracranial pressure and loss in sensory/motor function.

**Imaging Characteristics:** MRI is more sensitive than CT for the detection of brain metastasis.

## CT
- Shows multiple discrete lesions with variable density along the gray-white matter interface.
- Shows marked peripheral edema surrounding larger lesions.
- Post-contrast shows enhancement of the lesions.

## MRI
- Lesions are hypointense to isointense to brain parenchyma on T1-weighted images.
- T2-weighted images show the lesions and surrounding edema as high signal intensity.
- Post-contrast T1-weighted images demonstrate the lesions as hyperintense and the edema as hypointense.

**Treatment:** Usually patients with multiple metastatic lesions to the brain are treated with radiation therapy, while patients with a single metastatic lesion may undergo surgical removal of the lesion followed by radiation therapy.

**Prognosis:** Depends on the number and extent of metastatic lesions in the brain and if the patient has any evidence of other systemic cancer.

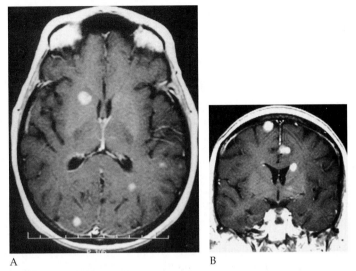

A                                          B

**FIGURE 1. Brain Metastasis.** Axial (A) and coronal (B) post contrast T1-weighted MRI shows multiple round contrast enhancing lesions involving gray and white matter as well as the gray-white matter junction.

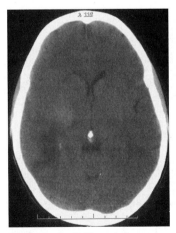

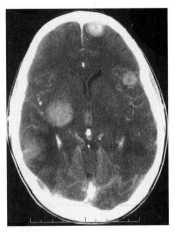

**FIGURE 2. Brain Metastasis.** Noncontrast CT of the head shows round high-density lesion in the region of the right basal ganglia with some mass effect on the right lateral ventricle.

**FIGURE 3. Brain Metastasis.** Post contrast CT of the head shows multiple round contrast enhancing lesions in the right parietal and left frontal lobes. There is edema with mass effect on the right lateral ventricle

# CRANIOPHARYNGIOMA

**Description:** Craniopharyngiomas are benign epithelial tumors that are almost always located in the suprasellar region and occasional in the intrasellar region.

**Etiology:** Craniopharyngiomas arise from squamous epithelial rests along the infundibulum of the hypophysis or Rathke's pouch.

**Epidemiology:** These tumors have a bimodal age distribution. More than half occur in children and young adults, while the second, smaller peak occurs in the fifth and sixth decade of life. Approximately 40 percent of craniopharyngiomas occur in children between the ages of 8 and 12 years. Males and females are affected equally.

**Signs and Symptoms:** Patients may present with visual symptoms, obstructive hydrocephalus, and endocrine dysfunction.

**Imaging Characteristics:** Small tumors are typically well-circumscribed, lobulated masses, while larger masses may be multicystic in appearance and invading the sella turcica. Craniopharyngiomas may present with calcification (90 percent), contrast enhance (90 percent), cystic (85 percent), and measure between 2 and 6 cm in size (75 percent).

## CT
- Lobulated solid and cystic suprasellar mass.
- Calcification seen in approximately 90 percent of pediatric tumors; and in adults 30 to 40 percent of adult tumors.
- Contrast enhancement of solid portions and periphery.

## MRI
- Appearance may be extremely variable, with most showing low signal on T1-weighted images and bright signal on T2-weighted images.
- Solid portions of the tumor usually enhance with contrast.
- Cystic areas may be hyperintense on T1-weighted images.

**Treatment:** Surgery is most commonly performed; however, the tumors may become so large that they are impossible to excise. Radiation therapy may also be used. Recurrence is common.

**Prognosis:** Surgical resection followed by radiation supports a 10-year survival rate of 78 percent.

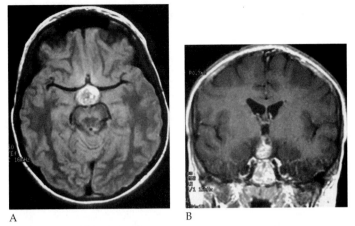

A                                      B

**FIGURE 1. Craniopharyngioma.** MRI FLAIR axial (A) and coronal (B) images demonstrate round high signal intense suprasellar mass.

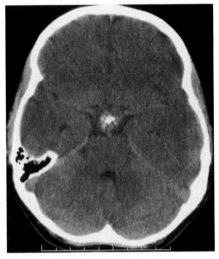

**FIGURE 2. Craniopharyngioma.** Noncontrast CT shows suprasellar calcifications.

# GLIOBLASTOMA MULTIFORME

**Description:** According to the WHO classification, a glioblastoma multiforme, also known as an astrocytoma grade IV tumor, is a rapid growing, highly malignant tumor. It is predominantly located in the intercerebral hemisphere although similar lesions may occur in the brainstem, cerebellum, or spinal cord. They spread by direct extension and can cross from one cerebral hemisphere to the other through connecting white matter tracts such as the corpus callosum.

**Etiology:** Unknown.

**Epidemiology:** The glioblastoma multiforme is the most common primary intracranial tumor. It typically appears between 45- and 60 years of age. Males are slightly more affected than females.

**Signs and Symptoms:** Patients may present with nausea and vomiting, headaches, papilledema, change in mental status, seizures, and speech and sensory disturbances.

**Imaging Characteristics:** These tumors are located in the white matter of the cerebral hemisphere, and will appear heterogeneous, with edema and mass effect.

### CT
- Noncontrast study shows an isodense to hypodense mass with surrounding edema.
- Nodular-rim enhancement with IV contrast demonstrates a necrotic tissue center.
- Edema is generally present.

### MRI
- T1-weighted images presents as mixed signal intensity.
- T2-weighted images demonstrate an increased signal (hyperintense) indicating a tumor and edema.
- T1-weighted contrast enhanced images will demonstrate nodular-rim enhancement, the edema. and necrotic tissue as hypointense.

**Treatment:** Surgical resection (if operable), radiation therapy and chemotherapy are currently the methods for treatment.

**Prognosis:** Poor prognosis. The survival rate for 1 year is approximately 50 percent, and 15 percent at 2 years.

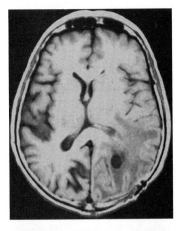

**FIGURE 1. Glioblastoma Multiforme.**
Noncontrast T1-weighted axial MRI shows low signal intensity lesion of the left occipital lobe with surrounding edema and mass effect on the left occipital lobe.

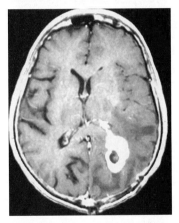

**FIGURE 2. Glioblastoma Multiforme.**
Post-contrast T1-weighted axial MRI shows irregular contrast enhancing mass in the left occipital lobe with surrounding edema and mass effect.

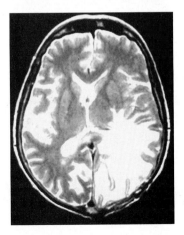

**FIGURE 3. Glioblastoma Multiforme.**
T2-weighted axial MRI shows diffuse increased signal intensity of the left parieto-occipital region representing edema.

# LIPOMA

**Description:** A benign fatty tumor.

**Etiology:** Unknown.

**Epidemiology:** Incidence of less then 1 percent of primary intracranial tumors. May appear at any age. Is usually located in the midline (80 -to 95 percent).

**Signs and Symptoms:** Asymptomatic, usually discovered as an incidental finding. Does not increase in size.

**Imaging Characteristics:**

**CT**
- Hypodense appearance. Does not enhance with contrast.

**MRI**
- Hyperintense on T1-weighted images.
- Hypointense on T2-weighted images.
- Fat suppression images will differentiate between fat and blood.

**Treatment:** No treatment may be required.

**Prognosis:** Unless the lipoma is positioned in a life-threatening location, the patient's prognosis is unaffected.

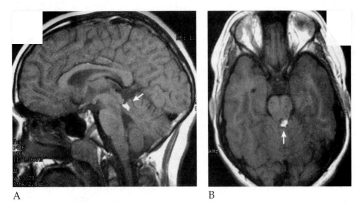

A                                                    B

**FIGURE 1. Lipoma.** T1-weighted sagittal (A) and axial (B) MR images show small high signal intense lesion just posterior to the tectum (*arrow*). This is consistent with a lipoma.

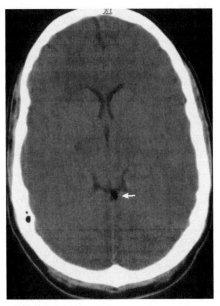

**FIGURE 2. Lipoma.** Axial noncontrast CT shows small low- density (fat density) lesion just posterior to the tectum (*arrow*).

# MEDULLOBLASTOMA

**Description:**  Medulloblastomas are rapid growing, highly malignant tumors arising in the posterior medullary velum.

**Etiology:**  Arises from the embryonal cell rests in the germinative zone of the posterior medullary velum, a midline structure that contributes to the roof of the fourth ventricle

**Epidemiology:**  These tumors are the most common posterior fossa neoplasm in pediatric patients and accounts for approximately 20 percent of all primary brain tumors in the pediatric population. There is a bimodal incidence, showing a major peak in children between 5 and 8 years of age and a second smaller peak between 20 and 30 years of age. Seen more than twice as often in males as in females.

**Signs and Symptoms:**  Patients may experience hydrocephalus- like signs and symptoms such as increased intracranial pressure (ICP), ataxia, or nystagmus. A herniation of the cerebellar tonsils can cause neck stiffness.

### Imaging Characteristics:

#### CT
- Noncontrast study is hyperdense in the midline displacing the fourth ventricle.
- IV contrast demonstrates enhancement of the mass.

#### MRI
- T1-weighted images range from hypointense to isointense to gray matter.
- Hyperintense on T2-weighted images.
- T1-weighted contrast enhanced images demonstrate irregular enhancement.

**Treatment:**  Methods of treatment may include surgical resection, radiation therapy, and multiagent chemotherapy.

**Prognosis:**  Good to poor prognosis depending on the patient's age, tumor location, and amount of tumor resected. Favorable prognostic factors include an age greater than 2 years, undisseminated local disease, and greater than 75 percent of the tumor resected.

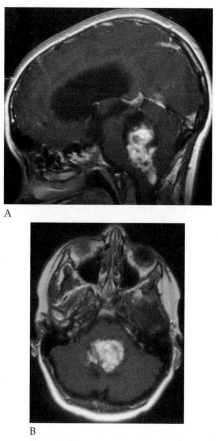

A

B

**FIGURE 1. Medulloblastoma.** Post contrast
T1-weighted sagittal (A) and axial (B) images
demonstrate irregular contrast enhancing
mass in the posterior fossa posterior to
the brain stem and obstructing the fourth
ventricle resulting in hydrocephalus.

# MENINGIOMA

**Description:** Meningiomas are the most common benign intracranial neoplasms, and the second most common primary tumor affecting the central nervous system. Meningiomas are characteristically a slow growing, usually highly vascular tumor occurring mainly along the meningeal vessels and superior longitudinal sinus. They invade the dura and skull and lead to erosion and thinning of the skull. In some cases, these tumors may also grow on the spine.

**Etiology:** Arises from the meninges.

**Epidemiology:** Meningiomas are primarily adult tumors. They account for approximately 20 percent of all primary brain tumors. The peak incidence is between 40 and 60 years of age. Females are slightly more affected than males by a ratio of 3:2. The majority of meningiomas (90 percent) are intracranial, and 90 percent of these are supratentorial.

**Signs and Symptoms:** The signs and symptoms a patient may present depends on the location and size of the tumor, however, headaches, seizures, nausea and vomiting and changes in mental status may be seen.

**Imaging Characteristics:**

**CT**
- Noncontrast study demonstrates a slightly hyperintense extraaxial mass.
- IV contrast study demonstrates marked enhancement.
- Calcification is seen in 20 to 25 percent of tumors.

**MRI**
- T1-weighted images demonstrate an isointense to slightly hypointense mass.
- T1-weighted images greatly enhance following gadolinium administration.
- T2-weighted images demonstrate a meningioma as isointense to slight hypointense.

**Treatment:** Surgical resection is used to remove this benign mass. Radiotherapy may be useful when complete surgical removal is not possible or the meningioma recurs.

**Prognosis:** Completely resected meningiomas provide an excellent prognosis with 10-year survival rate of 80 to 90 percent.

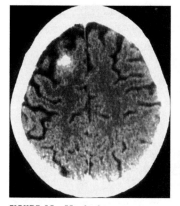

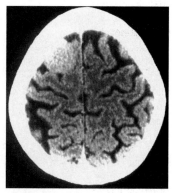

**FIGURE 1A. Meningioma.**
Noncontrast CT of brain shows a
meningioma in the right frontal
lobe with calcification.

**FIGURE 1B. Meningioma.**
Noncontrast CT shows round high
density mass over the convexity of
the right parietal lobe.

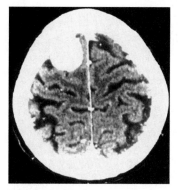

**FIGURE 1C. Meningioma.** Postcontrast CT image shows a round
markedly contrast enhancing mass
over the convexity of the right
parietal lobe.

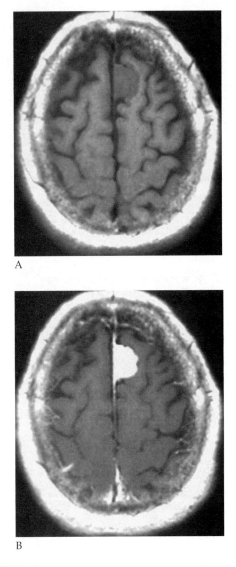

**FIGURE 2. Meningioma.** T1-weighted axial MR image shows an isointense left parasagittal meningioma (A) and post-contrast T1-weighted images in the, axial (B), coronal (C), and sagittal (D) planes, show marked enhancement.

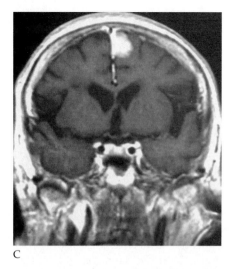

C

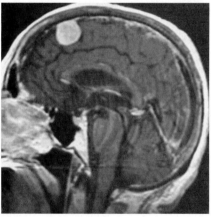

D

# PITUITARY ADENOMA

**Description:** Pituitary adenomas are also classified as either functioning or nonfunctioning depending on their ability to secret hormones.

**Etiology:** Although the exact cause is unknown, there is a predisposition that pituitary tumors are inherited through an autosomal dominant trait.

**Epidemiology:** Pituitary adenomas constitute 10 percent of all intracranial neoplasms and are the most common primary neoplasm found in the sellar region. They occur in both male and females equally during the third and fourth decades of life.

**Signs and Symptoms:** Patients may present with frontal headaches, visual symptoms, increased intracranial pressure, personality changes, seizures, rhinorrhea and pituitary apoplexy secondary to hemorrhagic infarction of the adenoma.

**Imaging Characteristics:** Adenomas that measure less than 10 mm are defined as microadenomas, while those measuring greater then 10 mm are defined as macroadenomas.

## CT
- Focal region of hypodensity within the gland.
- Following contrast enhancement, the tumor will be isodense to the normal pituitary gland.

## MRI
- T1-weighted images appear as a region of hypointensity within the gland.
- T1-weighted contrast enhanced images appear hyperintense.
- T1- and T2-weighted images may also show variable signal intensities within the mass.

**Treatment:** Methods may include transsphenoidal pituitary resection, cryohypophysectomy, pituitary irradiation or bromocriptine.

**Prognosis:** The patient's prognosis is good, depending on the extent the tumor spreads outside the sella turcica. It is a benign tumor.

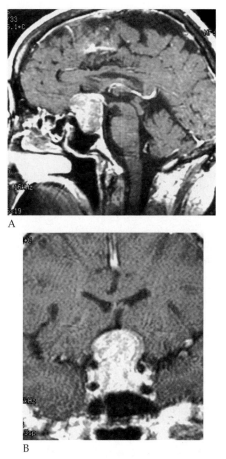

**FIGURE 1. Pituitary Adenoma.** Post-contrast T1-weighted sagittal (A) and coronal (B) MR images demonstrating a large contrast enhancing pituitary mass consistent with a macroadenoma.

# BRAIN
## CONGENITAL

# AGENESIS OF THE CORPUS CALLOSUM

**Description:** A partial or complete absence of the corpus callosum.

**Etiology:** Agenesis of the corpus callosum is caused by an insult that has occurred embryologically prior to the 10th week of gestation.

**Epidemiology:** Anomalies (agenesis) of the corpus callosum occur between 10 and 18 weeks of gestation. Males and females are equally affected.

**Signs and Symptoms:** Although patients may present asymptomatic, in many cases, there are developmental abnormalities present.

**Imaging Characteristics:** CT and MRI demonstrate an elevated third ventricle, noticeable separation of the lateral ventricles, partial or complete absences of the corpus callosum, and dysplasia of the cerebellum.

**Treatment:** There is no treatment for this condition, however, conditions such as hydrocephalus may require treatment

**Prognosis:** Depends other developmental abnormalities.

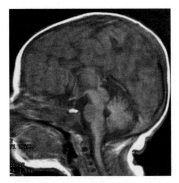

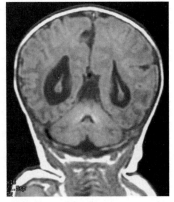

**FIGURE 1. Agenesis of the Corpus Callosum.** T1-weighted sagittal image shows complete absence of the corpus callosum with elevated third ventricle.

**FIGURE 2. Agenesis of the Corpus Callosum.** T1-weighted coronal image demonstrates separation of the lateral ventricles.

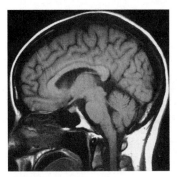

**FIGURE 3. Normal Corpus Callosum.** T1-weighted sagittal image shows a normal corpus callosum.

# DANDY-WALKER SYNDROME

**Description:**  Dandy-Walker syndrome is a noncommunicating type of hydrocephalus. It results from a partial dysgenesis of the vermis and a remnant fourth ventricle that communicates with a retrocerebellar cyst that is also known as a Blake's pouch (see "Hydrocephalus").

**Etiology:**  An atresia of the foramen of Magendie and foramina of Luschka of the fourth ventricle.

**Epidemiology:**  Represents approximately 2 percent of all cases of hydrocephalus. Occurs in one 1 per 25,000 to 30,000 births and is usually diagnosed by one 1 year of age. Males and females are equally affected. Associated with hydrocephalus in 80 percent of cases and agenesis of the corpus callosum in 20 percent of the cases.

**Signs and Symptoms:**  Related to hydrocephalus and other associated anomalies.

**Imaging Characteristics:**  Appears as a massively dilated fourth ventricle expanding into the posterior fossa demonstrating hydrocephalus. Both CT and MRI images demonstrate a massively dilated fourth ventricle, expanded posterior fossa with an inferior hypoplastic inferior vermis.

## CT
- Hypodense CSF filled space located in the posterior fossa involving the fourth ventricle.

## MRI
- Hypointense on T1-weighted images.
- Hyperintense on T2-weighted images.

**Treatment:**  Surgical intervention and shunting the excess CSF into the right atrium or the peritoneal cavity.

**Prognosis:**  Depends on other neurological abnormalities.

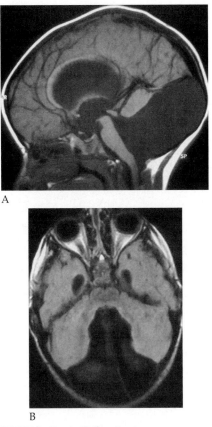

A

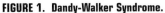

B

**FIGURE 1. Dandy-Walker Syndrome.**
T1-weighted sagittal (A) and axial (B) MR
images shows a massively dilated fourth
ventricle, expanded posterior fossa, high
insertion of the venous torcular, and
hypoplastic vermis in a complete Dandy-
Walker syndrome.

# ENCEPHALOCELE

**Description:** Encephaloceles result from a herniation of the brain or meninges, or both, through a skull defect. The hernia may be a small CSF-filled meningeal sac or a large cyst-like structure that may exceed the size of the head. It may be covered with skin and/or membrane of varying thickness, and may contain the pons, midbrain, and vermis structures. The herniated portion of the brain is nonfunctioning.

**Etiology:** Results from a congenital defect or a trauma opening in the skull.

**Epidemiology:** Newborns are mostly affected. Encephaloceles account for 10 to 20 percent of craniospinal malformations. The incidence rate is approximately 1 to 3 per 10,000 births. The skull defect is commonly found in the occipital region (71 percent), parietal region (10 percent) and throughout the skull base (18 percent).

**Signs and Symptoms:** Patients may present with hydrocephalus, developmental delay, motor weakness and/or spasticity, ataxia, mental retardation, microcephaly, seizures, and visual problems.

## Imaging Characteristics:

### CT
- Osseous defect is best evaluated with CT

### MRI
- Provides excellent delineation of the CSF and soft- tissue brain components of an encephalocele.

**Treatment:** In cases involving hydrocephalus, shunting CSF from the brain may be necessary.

**Prognosis:** The prognosis of fetuses with an encephalocele is variable depending on the presence of brain in the sac, hydrocephalus, and microcephaly. With brain involvement, the prognosis may be quite poor.

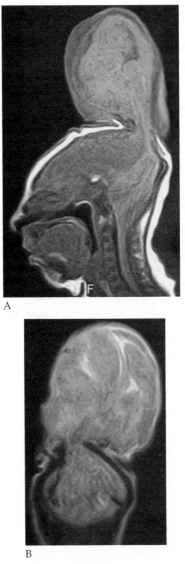

A

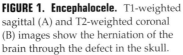

B

**FIGURE 1. Encephalocele.** T1-weighted sagittal (A) and T2-weighted coronal (B) images show the herniation of the brain through the defect in the skull.

# HYDROCEPHALUS

**Description:**  Hydrocephalus is an enlargement of the ventricular system of the brain also known in layman terms as "water on the brain.". There are two types of hydrocephalus: noncommunicating and communicating. Hydrocephalus may result from an excessive amount of cerebral spinal fluid production, inadequate reabsorption of CSF, or an obstruction of the flow of the CSF from one or more of the ventricles.

In the noncommunicating type of hydrocephalus, the flow of the (CSF) from the ventricular system into the subarachnoid space is obstructed by a mass-occupying lesion, congenital narrowing of the aqueduct of Sylvius, or associated with a meningomyelocele.

The communicating type of hydrocephalus may result from an overproduction of CSF in the choroid plexus, or inadequate reabsorption of CSF by the arachnoid villi.

**Note:**
1. In the Dandy-Walker syndrome, an atresia of the foramen of Magendie results in an enlarged fourth ventricle.
2. Normal pressure hydrocephalus typically affects adults with progressive dementia.

**Etiology:**  Hydrocephalus may result from: (1) an excessive amount of CSF production; (2) inadequate reabsorption of CSF by the arachnoid villi; or (3) an obstruction of the out flow of the CSF from one or more of the ventricles.

**Epidemiology:**  This congenital defect may also be associated with a history of a meningomyelocele.

**Signs and Symptoms:**  Patient may present with increase in the circumference of the head, behavioral changes such as irritability and lethargy, seizures and vomiting or a change in appetite.

**Imaging Characteristics:**  MRI is the better modality for the evaluation of hydrocephalus.

## CT
- Non-contrast study demonstrates enlarged ventricles (hypodense).

## MRI
- T1-weighted images demonstrate the enlarged CSF-filled ventricles as hypointense.

- T1-weighted contrast enhanced sequence should be performed to rule out intracranial mass if indicated.
- T2-weighted images demonstrate the enlarged CSF-filled ventricles as hyperintense

**Treatment:** Shunting the excess CSF into the right atrium or into the peritoneal cavity.

**Prognosis:** Good, following shunting procedure.

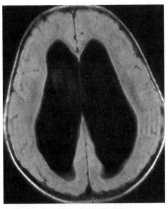

**FIGURE 1. Hydrocephalus.**
T1-weighted axial MRI shows markedly dilated lateral ventricles with low signal CSF.

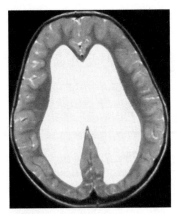

**FIGURE 2. Hydrocephalus.**
T2-weighted axial MRI shows high signal CSF of the markedly dilated lateral ventricles.

# BRAIN
## VASCULAR DISEASE

## ARTERIOVENOUS MALFORMATION

**Description:** An arteriovenous malformation (AVM) is the most common type of vascular malformation and is characterized by direct artery-to-vein communication without an intervening capillary bed.

**Etiology:** An AVM is a congenital lesion, which is the result of abnormal fetal development at approximately 3 weeks gestation.

**Epidemiology:** Males generally present during middle age and are slightly more affected than females. Between 80 and 90 percent are located in the cerebrum, and between 10 and 20 percent located in the posterior fossa.

**Signs and Symptoms:** Clinical presentation depends on the location and size of the AVM with most present between the second and third decade of life. By age 50, 80 to 90 percent are symptomatic. Hemorrhage will be present in approximately 50 percent of the cases. Other symptoms include seizures and headaches.

**Imaging Characteristics:** Appears as a collection of "worms."

### CT
- Isodense to slightly hyperdense without contrast enhancement.
- Calcification in 25 to 30 percent of lesions.
- Atrophy.
- Hyperdense serpentine-appearing vessels with contrast enhancement.

### MRI
- T1- and T2-weighted images demonstrate serpentine appearing vessels with signal variations (flow void) in the vessels.

**Treatment:** Depends on the age and general health of the patient. Endovascular embolization therapy, surgery intervention, stereotactic radiotherapy, or a combination of the above is useful in treating an AVM.

**Prognosis:** The mortality rate is approximately 10 percent when a hemorrhage is present.

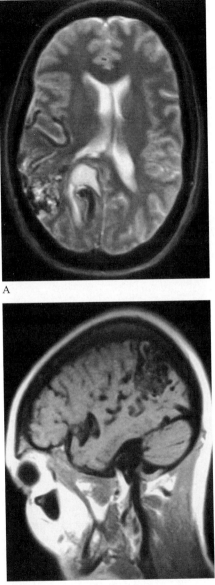

A

B

**FIGURE 1.  Arteriovenous Malformation.**
T1-weighted sagittal (A) and T2-weighted
axial (B) images demonstrate collection of
signal void worms in the right posterior
parietal and occipital lobes.

# INTRACRANIAL ANEURYSM

**Description:** An intracranial aneurysm is a localized dilation of a cerebral artery. The most common form is the berry aneurysm, a saclike outpouching usually arising from at an arterial junction in the circle of Willis. Cerebral aneurysms often rupture and result in a subarachnoid hemorrhage

**Etiology:** Weakening of the arterial wall may result from hemodynamic stresses. As an example, hypertension and atherosclerosis may restrict blood flow thus increasing blood pressure against an arterial wall, stretching it like an overblown balloon and making it likely to rupture. There is an increased incidence with polycystic kidney disease, aortic coarctation and family history.

**Epidemiology:** Incidence rate is slightly higher in women than men. The peak age of occurrence is between 40 and 60 years. Anterior circulation is affected 90 percent of the time, while the vertebrobasilar circulation affected only 10 percent.

**Signs and Symptoms:** Intracranial aneurysms may go undetected until they rupture, however, a very large **nonruptured** aneurysm can mimic the signs and symptoms of a tumor. If the aneurysm ruptures, they usually present as a subarachnoid hemorrhage. Signs and symptoms may vary depending on the location and severity of the ruptured aneurysm. Other common signs and symptoms may include headaches, nausea and vomiting, hemiparesis or motor deficit, nuchal rigidity, loss of consciousness, and coma.

**Imaging Characteristics:** Conventional angiography is the gold standard for the diagnosis of aneurysms.

## CT

- In patients with ruptured intracranial aneurysm, a noncontrast study demonstrates a subarachnoid hemorrhage in the basilar cisterns as hyperdense in approximately 95 percent of the cases.
- Contrast- enhanced CT may show very large aneurysm.

## MRI

- T1- and T2-weighted images appear with variable intensities (flow void).
- Magnetic resonance angiography (MRA) can diagnose most large aneurysms (>5 mm).

**Treatment:** Surgical intervention is best accomplished by a small metal clip or ligation around the neck of the aneurysm. Neuroradiologic intervention techniques also available for treatment of intracranial aneurysms include Guglielmi detachable (GD) coils.

**Prognosis:** In event that the aneurysm ruptures, the prognosis may be determined by the severity of the initial hemorrhage, rebleeding of the aneurysm, and vasospasm.

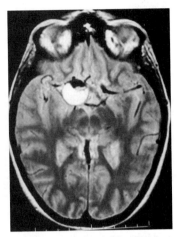

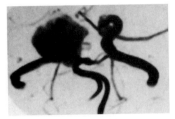

**FIGURE 1. Intracranial Aneurysm.** Axial MRA of the circle of Willis shows a large aneurysm of the right internal carotid artery.

**FIGURE 2. Intracranial Aneurysm.** Proton- density axial MRI shows a large mixed signal intensity aneurysm of the right internal carotid aneurysm.

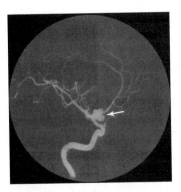

**FIGURE 3. Intracranial Aneurysm.** Oblique view of the right carotid arteriogram shows a large lobulated aneurysm (*arrow*) of the right internal carotid artery at its bifurcation.

# INTRACEREBRAL HEMORRHAGE (HEMORRHAGIC STROKE)

**Description:** Intracerebral hemorrhages (ICH) occur when blood escapes from a ruptured vessel in the brain.

**Etiology:** Results from a rupturing of a blood vessel, usually an artery, within the brain. Hemorrhagic infarcts are frequently associated with hypertension, arteriosclerosis or an aneurysm. Other factors may include trauma, neoplasms (primary or metastases) or drug use such as cocaine, amphetamine, and phenylpropanolamine.

**Epidemiology:** Approximately 20 percent of all strokes are hemorrhagic.

**Signs and Symptoms:** Patient may present with paralysis, motor weakness, headaches, or loss of consciousness.

**Imaging Characteristics:** CT is the modality of choice for the diagnosis of an intracranial hemorrhage.

## CT
- Hyperacute (less than 4 hours) hyperdense.
- Acute (24 to 72 hours) hyperdense.
- Early Subacute (4 to 7 days) hyperdense.
- Late Subacute (1 to 4 weeks) isodense.
- Chronic (2 weeks or more) hypodense.

## MRI

| Time | T1W1 | T2W1 | GRE |
|---|---|---|---|
| Acute (24 to 72 hours) | Isointense | Hypointense | Hypointense |
| Early Subacute (4 to 7 days) | Isointense to Hypointense | Hyperintense | Hypointense |
| Late Subacute (1 to 4 weeks) | Hyperintense | Hyperintense | Hypointense |
| Chronic (> 2 weeks) | Hypointense | Hypointense | Hypointense |

**Treatment:** Directed at reducing intracranial pressure (ICP) and controlling recurrent bleeding. Emergent surgery may be necessary to remove larger hematoma.

**Prognosis:** Depends on the location and severity of the hemorrhage.

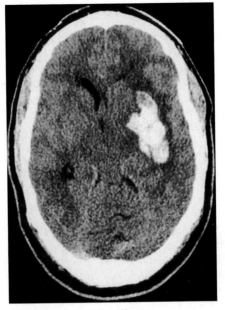

**FIGURE 1.  Intracerebral Hematoma.**
Noncontrast CT of the head shows a large
hematoma in the left basal ganglia with some
surrounding edema. There is compression of
the left lateral ventricle and some midline
shift to the right.

# ISCHEMIA STROKE: (CEREBROVASCULAR ACCIDENT)

**Description:** A cerebrovascular accident (CVA), or stroke, occurs as a result of ischemia or hemorrhage. Cerebral ischemia is a reduction in the regional or global blood flow to the brain.

**Etiology:** Thromboembolic disease, usually as a result of atherosclerosis, is the primary cause of ischemic cerebrovascular disease. The source of emboli may vary and arise from arterial stenosis and occlusion, atherosclerotic debris or from cardiac sources. Emboli from a cardiac source occur in approximately 15 to 20 percent of ischemic strokes.

**Epidemiology:** Approximately 80 to 85 percent of all strokes are ischemic. This is the third leading cause of death among Americans; following cardiovascular disease and cancer which are first and second, respectively. Males are affected approximately three times more frequently than females. People over older than 65 years of age are at a greater risk. Black men are 1.5 times more at risk for having a stroke than white men.

**Signs and Symptoms:** Depends on the etiology, location of the ischemia and the extent of damage to the brain cells.

**Imaging Characteristics:** MRI is more sensitive than CT, however noncontrast CT is more efficient for the diagnosis of an acute stroke to rule out hemorrhage.

## CT
- Is useful in establishing the presence or absence of a hemorrhage and therefore prescribing a thrombolytic or anticoagulant treatment.
- Acute stage: noncontrast study demonstrates a hyperdense middle cerebral artery, disappearing basal ganglia, and loss of insular cortex.
- Subacute stage: noncontrast study demonstrates wedge-shaped area of low density involving both gray and white matter.

## MRI
- Might identify approximately 80 percent of strokes during the initial 24 hours.
- Acute stage: vascular enhancement (slow flow) sign may be seen within 2 hours after ictus.

- Subacute stage: parenchymal enhancement may appear hyper-intense on T2-weighted images.
- Chronic stage: appears hypointense on T1-weighted images and hyperintense on T2-weighted images. Chances of malacia with brain volume loss.
- Diffusion-weighted imaging (DWI) is more sensitive in showing an infarct within a few hours, as an area of increased signal.

**Treatment:** Depending on the time of onset, thrombolytic therapy may be helpful if administered within the first 3 hours following the initial onset of an ischemic stroke. Other methods of treatment may include anticoagulant therapy such as the use of heparin and warfarin or the administration of calcium channel blocking drugs.

**Prognosis:** Depends on the severity of the stroke. There is a 50 percent mortality rate within the first 24 hours following a stroke. Strokes affecting the posterior circulation have a higher mortality rate, but usually make a better recovery than hemispheric strokes.

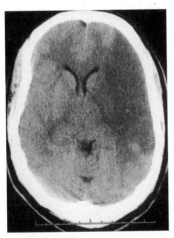

**FIGURE 1. Ischemic Stroke.**
Noncontrast CT demonstrates low-density area involving the left temporal and parietal lobes in the distribution of the left middle cerebral artery consistent with subacute infarct.

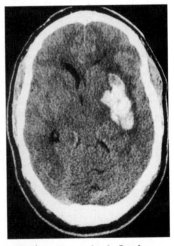

**FIGURE 2. Hemorrhagic Stroke.**
Noncontrast CT of the head shows a large hematoma in the left basal ganglia with some surrounding edema and compression of the left lateral ventricle and midline shift to the right.

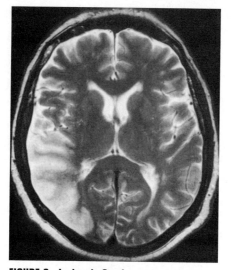

**FIGURE 3. Ischemic Stroke.** T2-weighted image demonstrates increased signal intensity of the cortex in the right posterior parietal lobe consistent with acute infarct.

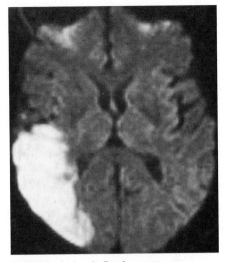

**FIGURE 4. Ischemic Stroke.** Diffusion-weighted image clearly shows the hyperintense right posterior parietal infarct.

# BRAIN
## INFECTION

# BRAIN ABSCESS

**Description:**  An intracranial abscess is a free or encapsulated collection of pus that usually is located in the frontal, temporal, or parietal lobes of the brain.

**Etiology:**  Usually occurs secondary to some other infection (e.g., otitis media, sinusitis, dental abscess, and mastoiditis). Other causes include subdural empyema, bacterial endocarditis, human immunodeficiency virus infection, bacteremia, pulmonary or pleural infection, abdominal/pelvic infections and open head injuries.

**Epidemiology:**  Males are 2:1 more likely to be affected than females. Brain abscesses can occur at any age, however, the median age is between 30 and 40.

**Signs and Symptoms:**  Patients may present with headaches, nausea and vomiting, change in mental status, afebrile or low-grade fever, seizures, and papilledema.

**Imaging Characteristics:**

### CT
- Hypodense-to-isodense on noncontrast study.
- Ring-like enhancement with contrast.
- Marked edema appearance surrounding the abscess

### MRI
- Hypointense to gray matter on T1-weighted images.
- Hyperintense to gray matter on T2-weighted images with surrounding edema.
- Ring-like enhancement following administration of contrast.

**Treatment:**  Antibiotics and possible surgical intervention are used in the treatment of brain abscesses.

**Prognosis:**  A survival rate of 80 percent or greater when diagnosed early.

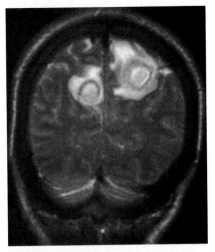

**FIGURE 1. Brain Abscess.** T2-weighted coronal image demonstrating round hyperintense lesions in bilateral occipital lobes with low signal peripheral rim. There is moderate surrounding edema.

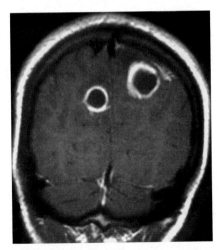

**FIGURE 2. Brain Abscess.** Postcontrast T1-weighted coronal image demonstrating ring-like contrast-enhancing lesions in the occipital lobes.

# CYSTICERCOSIS

**Description:** Cysticercosis is the most common parasitic infection of the central nervous system. Almost all cases of cysticercosis involve the brain.

**Etiology:** Results from the ingestion of ova of the pork tapeworm Taenia solium.

**Epidemiology:** Most common CNS parasitic infection worldwide. Endemic in Mexico, Central and South America, Eastern Europe, Africa, and parts of Asia. Most cases in developed countries occur in immigrants from endemic areas. CNS involvement occurs in 60 to 90 percent of infected patients.

**Signs and Symptoms:** Seizures are the most common seen in CNS involvement.

## Imaging Characteristics:

### CT
- Depicts spherical CSF-filled (hypodense) cysts.
- Ring-enhancing lesions on contrast studies.
- May show calcified lesions.

### MRI
- The cyst appears hypointense on T1-weighted sequences.
- A scolex (the attachment organ of a tapeworm) may be seen in the center of the cyst on T1-weighted images.
- Ring-like enhancement of the cyst on T1-weighted contrast studies.
- Edema and the cyst appear hyperintense on T2-weighted images.

**Treatment:** An anthelmintic agent such as praziquantel or albendazole. These agents are used to kill the parasite. Surgical intervention may be required to remove intraventricular cysts, ventricular shunting, or both.

**Prognosis:** Morbidity usually results from dying larvae that bring about an intense inflammatory response.

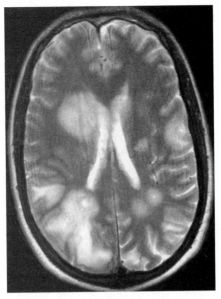

**FIGURE 1. Cysticercosis.** T2-weighted MR axial image demonstrates a bright signal at the site of the lesions and surrounding edema.

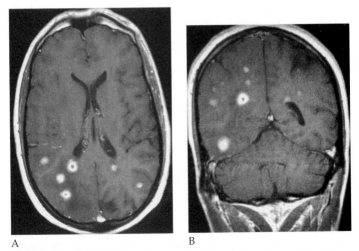

A                                        B

**FIGURE 2. Cysticercosis.** MRI postcontrast T1-weighted axial (A) and coronal (B) images demonstrate multiple small, round, enhancing lesions in the bilateral occipital lobes with surrounding low signal edema.

# MULTIPLE SCLEROSIS

**Description:** Multiple sclerosis (MS) is a demyelinating disease that is characterized by multiple inflammatory plaques of demyelination involving the white matter tracts of the central nervous system (brain and spine). This progressive disease is further characterized by the destruction of the lipid and protein layer called the myelin sheath that insulates the axon part of the nerve cell. The areas of demyelination are commonly referred to as "plaques." Multiple sclerosis may go through periods of exacerbation and remission.

**Etiology:** Unknown, however, theories suggest a slow-acting viral infection and an autoimmune response. Other theories suggest environmental and genetic factors.

**Epidemiology:** Females are slightly more affected than males at a ratio of 3:2. The incidence rate is between 18 and 50 years of age. In addition, MS occurs most often in people of European descent, less often in Asians, and rarely in black Africans.

**Signs and Symptoms:** Patients may present with paresthesia or abnormal sensations in the extremities or on one side of the face; numbness, tingling, or a "pins and needles" type of feeling; muscle weakness; vertigo; visual disturbances, such as nystagmus, diplopia (double vision), and partial blindness; extreme emotional changes; ataxia; abnormal reflexes; and difficulty in urinating.

**Imaging Characteristics:** MRI is the imaging modality of choice for diagnosis of multiple sclerosis.

### MRI
- T1-weighted images appear isointense to hypointense.
- Proton density weighted images appear hyperintense.
- T2-weighted images appear hyperintense.
- FLAIR images are very useful and show hyperintense white matter lesions
- Active plaques may show contrast enhancement.

**Treatment:** There is no specific treatment for MS.
- Corticosteroids and other drugs, however, are used to treat the symptoms.
- Physical therapy may help to postpone or prevent specific disabilities.

**Prognosis:** The course of the multiple sclerosis disease process is varied and unpredictable.

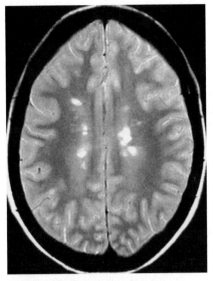

**FIGURE 1. Multiple Sclerosis.** MR proton-density axial image shows ovoid hyperintense lesions (Dawson fingers) in the centrum semiovale bilaterally.

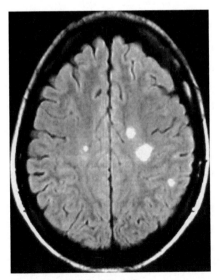

**FIGURE 2. Multiple Sclerosis.** Postcontrast T1-weighted axial MR shows enhancement of active multiple sclerosis plaques.

# BRAIN
## PHAKOMATOSIS

## STURGE-WEBER SYNDROME

**Description:** Sturge-Weber syndrome (encephalotrigeminal angiomatosis) is a congenital disorder characterized by localized atrophy and calcification of the cerebral cortex with an ipsilateral port-wine–colored facial nevus in the area of the trigeminal nerve distribution.

**Etiology:** Hereditary disorder attributed to autosomal dominant and autosomal recessive patterns.

**Epidemiology:** Incidence is 1 per 1000 patients in mental institutions.

**Signs and Symptoms:** Patients may present with port-wine stain, seizure disorder, hemiatrophy, hemianopsia, mental retardation, and glaucoma.

### Imaging Characteristics:

#### CT
- Cerebral atrophy may be seen.
- Calcified areas of the brain which appear hyperdense.

#### MRI
- Cerebral atrophy is best seen on T1-weighted images.
- Lower (hypointense) signal may be present in calcified areas of the brain.
- FLAIR images are used to demonstrate leptomeningeal (pia mater and arachnoid) abnormality as a hyperintense signal.

**Treatment:** Symptomatic treatment for the above-mentioned conditions.

**Prognosis:** Most cases are considered to be mild and life expectancy is usually normal.

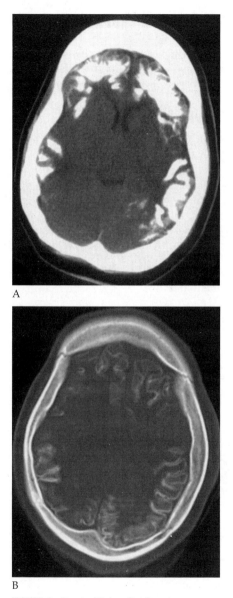

A

B

**FIGURE 1.  Sturge-Weber Syndrome.**
Noncontrast CT images of the brain (A)
and bone window (B) demonstrate bilateral
frontal and parietal cortical calcifications.

# VON HIPPEL-LINDAU DISEASE

**Description:** An autosomal dominant (hereditary) condition characterized by angiomas of the retina and cerebellum, visceral cysts and malignancies, seizures and mental retardation.

**Etiology:** Hereditary disorder.

**Epidemiology:** Prevalence is estimated at 1 in 35,000 to 40,000 population. There is no predilection towards males or females.

**Signs and Symptoms:** Patients typically become symptomatic in their third or fourth decade of life. Characterized by retinal angiomas, hemangioblastomas of the cerebellum and spinal cord, cystic disease of the kidney, pancreas, and liver, and a risk of malignancy involving the kidneys, adrenal glands, or pancreas. Patients may experience seizures and mental retardation.

## Imaging Characteristics:

### MRI
- Tumors within the CNS appear as isointense to hypointense on T1-weighted images.
- T2-weighted images present the tumors as hyperintense.
- T1-weighted images with contrast demonstrate the tumor as hyperintense (the most sensitive means of detecting the CNS tumor).

**Treatment:** Symptomatic treatment for the above mentioned conditions and surgical intervention of tumors where and when appropriate.

**Prognosis:** Varies depending on degree of symptoms and if cancer is detected. There is no known cure for this hereditary disease. Death is usually associated with complications of brain tumors or renal cancer.

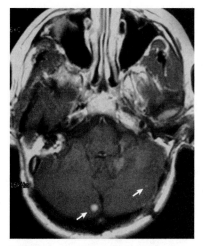

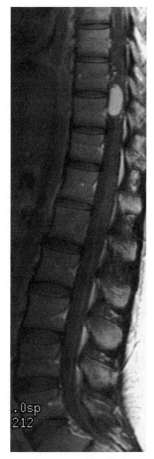

**FIGURE 1. von Hippel-Lindau Disease.**
Postcontrast T1-weighted axial MR
image of the brain shows round
contrast enhancing lesions (*arrows*)
located bilaterally in the cerebellar
hemispheres consistent with
hemangioblastomas.

**FIGURE 2. von Hippel-Lindau Disease.**
Postcontrast T1-weighted sagittal MR
image of the thoracolumbar spine
demonstrating an oval contrast
enhancing intradural/extramedullary
mass at T9 and T10 consistent with a
hemangioblastoma.

# BRAIN
## TRAUMA

## Epidural Hematoma

**Description:** An epidural hematoma is a mass of blood frequently formed as a result a trauma to the head. Although mostly arterial in origin and located between the skull and the dura mater in the temporoparietal region, epidural hematomas are strongly associated with a linear skull fracture, which can cause a tear of the middle meningeal artery. Less common in occurrence are venous epidural hematomas, which typically occur in the posterior fossa or adjacent to the occipital lobes of the cerebrum.

**Etiology:** Usually the result of blunt trauma to the head with a tearing of the middle meningeal artery causing hemorrhaging into the epidural space.

**Epidemiology:** Individuals who have experienced blunt trauma to the head are at risk.

**Signs and Symptoms:** Patients may present with loss of consciousness (LOC), hemiparesis, headaches, dilated pupils, increased intracranial pressure (ICP), nausea and vomiting, dizziness, convulsions, and decerebrate rigidity.

**Imaging Characteristics:** Appears to be biconvex in shape and displacing the brain away from the skull. Noncontrast CT is the imaging modality of choice.

### CT
- Underlying fracture.
- Acute stage hemorrhage will appear hyperdense.
- Subacute stage hemorrhage will appear isodense.
- Chronic stage may appear as hypodense.

### MRI
- Subacute stage appears hyperintense on T1- and T2-weighted images.
- Acute stage hemorrhage will appear isointense on T1-weighted images and hypointense on T2-weighted images.

**Treatment:** Surgical emergency is required to remove the accumulated blood.

**Prognosis:**  With early diagnosis and treatment, prognosis is good; however, with large epidural hematomas, the outcome may result in neurologic deficit.

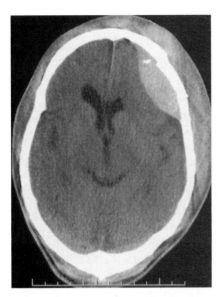

**FIGURE 1.  Epidural Hematoma.**  Noncontrast CT shows typical biconvex hyperdense acute left frontal epidural hematoma with mass effect on the left frontal lobe. ·

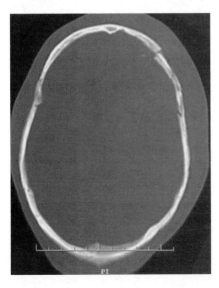

**FIGURE 2.  Epidural Hematoma.**  Noncontrast CT on the same patient shows left frontal skull fracture.

# Subarachnoid Hemorrhage

**Description:** A subarachnoid hemorrhage (SAH) involves the escape of blood into the subarachnoid space especially the basal cisterns and into the cerebral spinal fluid (CSF) pathways.

**Etiology:** Subarachnoid hemorrhages occur most often as a result of a ruptured saccular (Berry) aneurysm. Other causes may include intracranial arteriovenous malformations (AVM), hypertension or traumatic injury to the head.

**Epidemiology:** Approximately 11 of 100,000 people are affected annually. Traumatic incidents may occur at any age. The maximal incidence rate for a subarachnoid hemorrhage is in the fourth and fifth decade of life.

**Signs and Symptoms:** Headaches are the most common symptoms associated with SAH. Other complications may include loss of consciousness and focal neurologic deficits.

**Imaging Characteristics:** Noncontrast CT is the modality of choice for diagnosis of a subarachnoid hemorrhage.

## CT
- Noncontrast exam reveals high-density acute blood present in the subarachnoid spaces (e.g., basilar cisterns and sylvian fissures).

## MRI
- MRI is not suitable for imaging most situations.
- FLAIR images are the most sensitive.
- FLAIR images show blood as hyperintensity in the subarachnoid space (CSF normally is nulled and therefore not visible).
- Magnetic resonance angiography (MRA) is useful to diagnose most large aneurysms (>5 mm).
- Conventional T1- and T2-weighted images are not very useful.
- Conventional angiography is the gold standard for the diagnosis of cerebral aneurysms.

**Treatment:** Treat the underlying aneurysm by placing a small metal clip or ligation around the neck of the aneurysm. Neuroradiologic intervention techniques also available for treatment of intracranial aneurysms include GD coils. Prevent complications of a SAH (i.e., vasospasms, rebleeding and hydrocephalus).

**Prognosis:** Varies depending on the severity of the initial hemorrhage, possibility of rebleeding, and vasospasm.

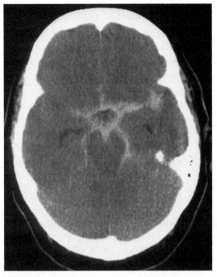

**FIGURE 1. Subarachnoid Hemorrhage.**
Noncontrast axial CT demonstrates blood in
the basilar cisterns as will as sylvian fissures.

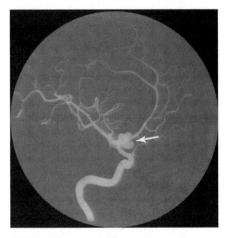

**FIGURE 2. Intracranial Aneurysm.** Oblique
view of the right carotid arteriogram shows a
large lobulated aneurysm (*arrow*) of the right
internal carotid artery at its bifurcation.

# Subdural Hematoma

**Description:** A subdural hematoma (SDH) is a collection of venous blood located between the dura mater and the arachnoid membrane (subdural space). A subdural hematoma usually develops as a result of the head hitting an immovable object. Though SDHs occur as a result of trauma, seldom are they associated with a skull fracture.

**Etiology:** A subdural hematoma is usually the result of the head striking an immovable object. High-speed acceleration- or deceleration-related head injuries could result in the tearing of the veins between the cerebral cortex and the dural veins. May also result from birth trauma or child abuse.

**Epidemiology:** Individuals who have experienced blunt trauma to the head are at risk, even though symptoms may not arise immediately. There are three time intervals between trauma and the onset of clinical symptoms. These time intervals vary from (1) 24 to 48 hours after injury is defined as acute; (2) between 48 hours and 2 weeks as subacute; and (3) 7 to 10 days as chronic.

**Signs and Symptoms:** Patients may present with headaches, a change in mental status, motor and sensory deficits, an increase in intracranial pressure, and possible deterioration of the neurologic status.

**Imaging Characteristics:** CT is the preferred modality for the diagnosis of acute SDH, where as MRI is more sensitive for a subacute or chronic SDH. Subdural hematomas typically are crescentic shaped, conforming to the contour of the cranium's inner table. They may extend into the interhemispheric or tentorial subdural space.

## CT
- Acute stage appears hyperdense.
- Subacute stage appears isodense.
- Chronic stage appears hypodense.

## MRI
- Acute stage appears hypointense to isointense on T1-weighted images and hypointense on T2-weighted images.
- Subacute stage appears hyperintense on T1-weighted images and hypointense on T2-weighted images.
- Chronic stage appears with a higher signal (intermediate) than CSF on T1-weighted images and hyperintense on T2-weighted images.

**Treatment:** A subdural hematoma may be drained through a burr hole or may require a craniotomy to drain the accumulated blood.

**Prognosis:** The mortality rates for acute and chronic subdural hematomas are greater than 50 percent and less than 10 percent, respectively. Most patients resume preoperative functional status. Outcome is highly dependent on the presurgical neurologic status.

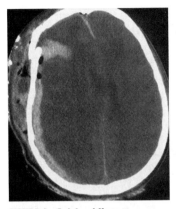

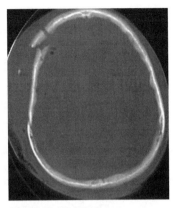

**FIGURE 1. Subdural Hematoma.** Noncontrast axial CT demonstrates a crescentic high-density acute right subdural hematoma in the right parietal and occipital region with mass effect on the right lateral ventricle and midline shift to the left. There is also a right frontal lobe hematoma (intracerebral). There is also a fracture of the right frontal bone as well as pneumocephalus.

**FIGURE 2. Skull Fracture.** Bone window setting of an axial CT shows a skull fracture (right frontal bone). There is air (pneumocephalus) in the subdural space.

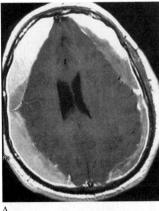

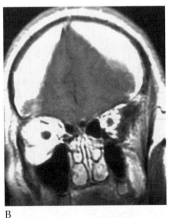

A                                    B

**FIGURE 3. Subdural Hematoma.** Noncontrast T1-weighted axial (A) and coronal (B) MR images demonstrate large bilateral, mostly high signal, subacute subdural hematomas.

# SPINE

## CONGENITAL

# ARNOLD-CHIARI MALFORMATION

**Description:** Arnold-Chiari malformations consist of a spectrum of congenital anomalies that affect the hindbrain. They are characterized by a downward elongation of the brainstem (medulla oblongata), cerebellum (cerebellar tonsils), and the fourth ventricle into the cervical portion of the spinal cord. Arnold-Chiari malformations are categorized into three types.

In an Arnold-Chiari type I, the cerebellar tonsils alone are displaced 5 to 6 mm below the foramen magnum. There is no hydrocephalus involved and the fourth ventricle remains in its normal location. A syringohydromyelia (syrinx) of the cervical spinal cord may be seen. This may be associated with Klippel-Feil syndrome.

In an Arnold-Chiari type II, the cerebellar tonsils and vermis of the fourth ventricle, cerebellum, and medulla oblongata have herniated down through the foramen magnum into the cervical spinal canal. Obstruction of the fourth ventricle results in hydrocephalus. This type is associated with myelomeningocele and agenesis of the corpus callosum.

An Arnold-Chiari type III malformation is characterized by displacement of the cerebellum meninges, and sometimes the brainstem, into an encephalocele. Encephaloceles results from a herniation of the brain or meninges, or both, through a skull defect. Characteristics seen in type II Arnold-Chiari malformations may be present. It occurs in approximately 1 in 4000 to 5000 deliveries.

**Etiology:** Although there are several theories of the cause of this malformation, the one that is generally accepted is that the posterior fossa is too small, causing a herniation of the brainstem and cerebellar tonsils through the foramen magnum into the upper cervical spinal canal.

**Epidemiology:** Type I Arnold-Chiari malformations are found more often in adults (incidentally by MRI) than in children. There does not seem to be any gender preference.

**Signs and Symptoms:** Hydrocephalus and developmental defects may be seen early on in infants. Young adults may be asymptomatic until neurologic deficits such as craniocervical junction abnormalities (e.g., progressive ataxia) occur.

**Imaging Characteristics:**  MRI is the modality of choice for diagnosing this disorder.

## CT
- The effectiveness of demonstrating this anomaly with CT is limited because of the bony surroundings and axial imaging.

## MRI
- T1- and T2-weighted pulse sequences will demonstrate the downward herniation of the cerebellar tonsils through the foramen magnum into the upper cervical canal.
- Associated findings may include syringomyelia and hydrocephalus.
- This malformation is best seen on sagittal images.

**Treatment:**  Surgery intervention may be used to decompress the posterior fossa. Shunt placement is used to treat hydrocephalus.

**Prognosis:**  Depends on the type, age of the patient when diagnosed, and extent of other related developmental defects. The prognosis for infants may be worse than for adults.

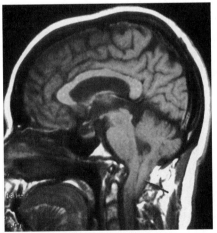

**FIGURE 1.  Arnold-Chiari Malformation.**
T1-weighted sagittal image demonstrates downward herniation of the cerebellar tonsils (*arrow*) through the foramen magnum into the upper cervical spinal canal with compression of the medulla oblongata.

# SYRINGOMYELIA/HYDROMYELIA

**Description:** Syringomyelia refers to any fluid-filled cavity within the spinal cord. A cavity in the cord may be caused by central canal dilatation (hydromyelia) or a cavity eccentric to the central canal (syrinx). It is difficult to differentiate between these two entities.

**Etiology:** Approximately 50 percent of syringomyelias are congenital (Chiari malformation). Acquired cases are the result of intramedullary tumors, trauma, infarction, and hemorrhage. In some cases, there is no known cause.

**Epidemiology:** Approximately 90 percent occur in association with an Arnold-Chiari type I malformation, but also may include, myelomeningocele, basilar skull impression (platybasia), atresia of the foramen of Magendie, or Dandy-Walker cysts.

**Signs and Symptoms:** Depends on the extent of the syrinx. The patient may experience sensory loss (loss of pain and temperature), muscle atrophy (lower neck, shoulders, arms and hands), and thoracic scoliosis.

**Imaging Characteristics:** MRI is the modality of choice for the diagnosis of syringomyelia.

## CT
- Postmyelogram CT demonstrates a contrast filled syrinx surrounded by the hypodense spinal cord.

## MRI
- Signal intensity of a syrinx may be isointense to CSF on T1-weighted images.
- Signal intensity of a syrinx would be isointense to CSF on T2-weighted images.

**Treatment:** Surgical drainage of the syrinx is the suggestive treatment.

**Prognosis:** Variable, depending on the extent of the syrinx.

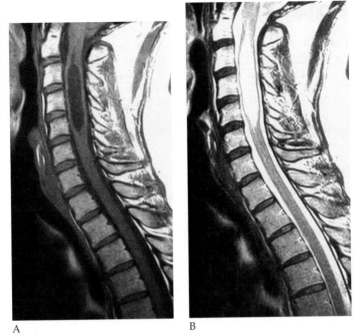

A                                    B

**FIGURE 1. Syringohydromyelia.** Sagittal T1- (A) and T2-weighted (B) MR images of the cervical spine show CSF signal intensity (low on the T1-weighted image and high on T2-weighted image) area within the spinal cord consistent with syringomyelia.

# TETHERED CORD

**Description:** A tethered cord is a condition in which the conus medullaris is prevented from ascending to its usual position at the level of L1–L2. It is tethered at an abnormally low position by a tight, short, thickened filum terminale, fibrous bands, intradural lipoma, or some other intradural abnormality.

**Etiology and Epidemiology:** This congenital abnormality is seen in neonates.

**Signs and Symptoms:** Patient presents with muscle weakness, abnormal lower limb reflexes, bowel and bladder dysfunction, back pain, and scoliosis.

**Imaging Characteristics:** MRI is the imaging modality of choice for the diagnosis of a tethered cord.

### MRI
- Tip of the conus medullaris is below the level of L2.
- T1-weighted axial shows a thickened (>2 mm in diameter) filum terminale.
- The conus medullaris may be tethered by spina bifida occulta and/or intradural lipoma (posteriorly displaced by fat), glial cells and collagen.

**Treatment:** Surgery in infancy or early childhood is required to prevent progressive neurologic deficit.

**Prognosis:** Depends on the extent of the tethered cord and age of the child at the time of diagnosis and treatment.

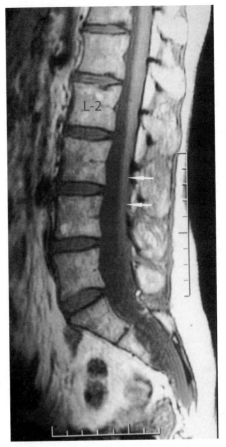

**FIGURE 1. Tethered Cord.** T1-weighted sagittal MR image shows the conus medullaris *(arrows)* to be below the level of L2.

# SPINE
## DEGENERATIVE

# HERNIATED DISK

**Description:** A herniated disk is also referred to as a ruptured or protruded disk. A herniated disk occurs when part or the entire nucleus pulposus (the soft, gelatinous, central portion of an intervertebral disk) is forced through the disk's weakened or torn outer ring (annulus fibrosus). This extruded herniated disk may impinge upon spinal nerve roots as they exit from the spinal canal, or on the spinal cord itself.

**Etiology:** Herniated disks may result from severe trauma or strain, or may be related to intervertebral disk degeneration. In older patients with degenerative disk disease, minor trauma may cause herniation.

**Epidemiology:** Approximately 90 percent of herniated disks occur in the lumbosacral spine, with the majority of these occurring at L5–S1, and the rest at either L4–L5 or L3–L4. A small percent of herniated disks involve the cervical spine, with the majority of these being at C5–C6 and C6–C7. Only 1 to 2 percent of herniated disks occur in the thoracic spine.

**Signs and Symptoms:** Patients with lumbosacral herniated disks present with low back pain, radiating to the buttocks, legs, and feet, usually unilaterally. Sensory and motor loss, muscle weakness, and atrophy of the leg muscles may be experienced if a lumbar spinal nerve root is compressed. Cervical disk herniations presents with pain in the neck and upper extremities, as well as weakness and neurological deficits, such as muscle spasms, numbness, and tingling are common symptoms.

**Imaging Characteristics:** As a result of excellent soft-tissue resolution and multiplanar imaging, MRI is the imaging modality of choice for diagnosing herniated disc.

### MRI and CT
- Demonstrate disc degeneration.
- Herniated disc usually lateralized to one side, compressing the thecal sac and nerve root.
- Free disc fragments may migrate superiorly or inferiorly.

**Treatment:** Conservative treatment consists of bed rest, heat, exercise, and medication, ranging from antiinflammatory drugs to muscle relaxants. Patients not responding to conservative treatment may require surgical intervention.

**Prognosis:** Prognosis is very mixed, dependent on the severity of damage, the quality and skill of surgical intervention, the age, size and weight of the patient, and whether there is a physically active or sedentary lifestyle.

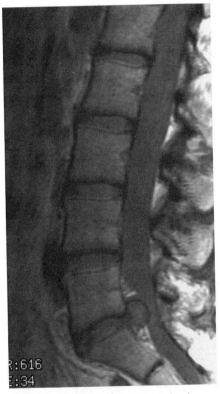

**FIGURE 1. Herniated Disc.** T1-weighted sagittal MR image shows herniated disc at the L5–S1 level.

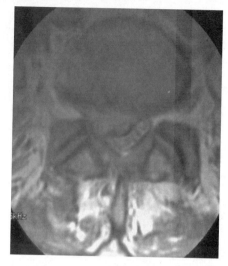

**FIGURE 2. Herniated Disc.** T1-weighted axial MR image demonstrates right-sided herniated disk at the L5–S1 level compressing the right side of the thecal sac and nerve root.

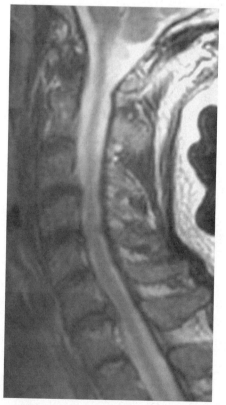

**FIGURE 3. Herniated Disc.** T1-weighted sagittal MR images show herniated disc at the C6–C7 level.

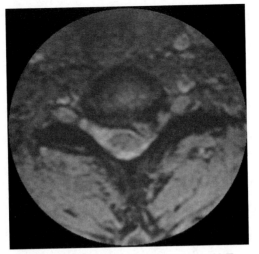

**FIGURE 4. Herniated Disc.** T1-weighted axial MR image demonstrates left sided herniated disc at the C6–C7 level with encroachment of the left side of the spinal canal and left neural foramen.

# SPINAL STENOSIS

**Description:** Spinal stenosis may be defined as the narrowing of the spinal canal and lateral recesses as a result of progressive degenerative disease of the disk, bone, and ligament. Problems arise when the spinal canal and cord are constricted. Mostly involves the cervical and lumbar spine.

**Etiology:** Spinal stenosis may be categorized as either congenital (developmental) or acquired. Congenital spinal stenosis may be caused by achondroplasia or anomaly, or it may be idiopathic. Acquired central spinal stenosis may result from several manifestations including degenerative disk disease, ligamentum flavum hypertrophy, spondylolisthesis, bulging disk, and trauma.

**Epidemiology:** Most commonly found in the cervical and lumbar spine.

**Signs and Symptoms:** When the cervical portion of the spine is involved, the patient may present with a radiculopathy, myelopathy, or neck or shoulder pain. If the lumbar spine is affected, the patient may present with a limping type of gait (neurogenic or spinal claudication), low back pain, or paresthesia of the lower extremities.

**Imaging Characteristics:** MRI is the modality of choice for diagnosing spinal stenosis. CT following myelography is the next best choice for imaging spinal stenosis.

## MRI and CT
- Narrowing of the spinal canal, lateral recess, and neural foramen.
- Bulging discs.
- Hypertrophy of facet joints and ligamentum flavum.
- Spondylolisthesis.
- Compression of the thecal sac and nerve roots.

**Treatment:** Surgical intervention may be considered.

**Prognosis:** This condition is progressive.

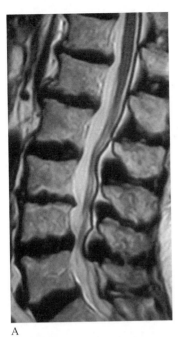

A

**FIGURE 1. Spinal Stenosis.** T2-weighted sagittal (A) and axial (B) MR images of the lumbar spine demonstrate narrowing of spinal canal secondary to bulging disc and hypertrophy of the facet and ligamentum flavum mostly at the L4–L5 level.

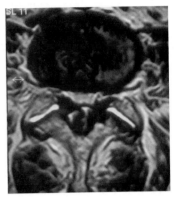

B

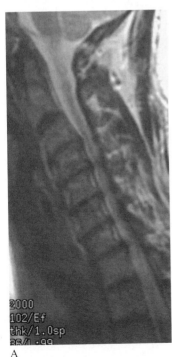

A

**FIGURE 2. Spinal Stenosis.** T2-weighted sagittal (A) and GRE axial (B) images of the cervical spine demonstrate narrowing of the spinal canal between C3–C7 secondary to bulging discs and/or posterior osteophytes. There is mild compression of the spinal cord.

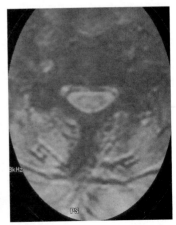

B

# SPONDYLOLISTHESIS

**Description:** Spondylolisthesis is the displacement or slippage, either anterior or posterior, of a vertebra over an inferior vertebra (usually the fifth lumbar vertebra over the sacrum, or the fourth lumbar vertebra over the fifth), causing a misalignment of the vertebral column. Type I involves a 25 percent vertebral displacement over the vertebra that is immediately inferior to it; type II involves a 50 percent vertebral displacement, and type III involves a 75 percent vertebral displacement over the inferior vertebra. Type IV involves anything over a 75 percent vertebral displacement over the inferior vertebra.

**Etiology:** Spondylolisthesis may result from acute trauma, or congenital or acquired fibrous defects in the pars interarticularis (spondylolysis), or as a result of spinal instability caused by degenerative changes involving the disk and facet joints.

**Epidemiology:** Spondylolisthesis occurs in 60 percent of patients with spondylolysis, which occurs in approximately 5 percent of the population. The L5–S1 interspace accounts for 90 percent of the cases of spondylolisthesis, with the majority of those cases being anterior displacement of the L5 vertebra. The L4–L5 interspace accounts for approximately 10 percent of spondylolisthesis cases, with most involving anterior slippage of L4 vertebra. Cervical spondylolisthesis comprises less than 1 percent of all cases.

**Signs and Symptoms:** Patients may present with low back pain and/or stiffness, and loss of function. Tight hamstrings may force the patient to walk with the knees bent and a short stride, causing poor posture or unusual gait.

**Imaging Characteristics:** Plain films are usually sufficient to make the diagnosis.

## CT
- Sagittal reformatted images demonstrate a shifting of a vertebra over an inferior vertebra.
- Shows pars interarticularis defects (spondylolysis).

## MRI
- Shows forward slippage of one vertebra over another. Best seen on a sagittal image.
- Shows other associated findings (e.g., degenerative disk disease and spinal stenosis).

**Treatment:** Conservative treatment is usually initiated to treat the patient's symptoms. Surgery may be indicated in symptomatic patients who do not respond to conservative treatment.

**Prognosis:** May vary depending on the type and other associated findings

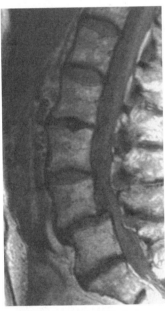

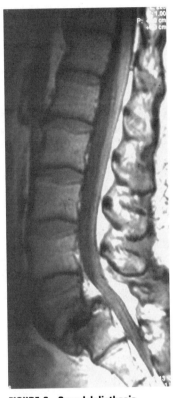

**FIGURE 1. Spondylolisthesis Grade I.** Sagittal T1-weighted MR image of the lumbar spine demonstrate mild forward displacement of the L4 vertebral body over L5. This is consistent with grade I spondylolisthesis. Degenerative changes of L4–L5 and L5–S1 discs noted.

**FIGURE 2. Spondylolisthesis Grade II.** T1-weighted sagittal image demonstrates a forward displacement of the L5 vertebral body over S1 consistent with a grade II spondylolisthesis. Note the degenerative changes of the L5–S1 disk.

# SPINE

## INFECTION

# Multiple Sclerosis: (Spinal Cord)

**Description:** Multiple sclerosis (MS) is a demyelinating disease affecting the spinal cord (see "Brain: Infection: Multiple Sclerosis"). The areas of demyelination are commonly referred to as "plaques." Multiple sclerosis may go through periods of exacerbation and remission.

**Etiology:** The exact cause of multiple sclerosis is unknown, however, theories suggest a slow-acting viral infection and an autoimmune response. Other theories suggest environmental and genetic factors.

**Epidemiology:** Multiple sclerosis commonly involves the spinal cord. Rarely is MS seen in children and older adults. Females are slightly more affected than males.

**Signs and Symptoms:** Patient presents with focal neurologic attacks, progressive deterioration and ultimately permanent neurologic dysfunction. Other complications include sensory and motor dysfunction.

**Imaging Characteristics:** MRI is the imaging modality of choice for the diagnosis of multiple sclerosis in the spinal cord.

**MRI**
- T1-weighted images are useful to evaluate the spinal cord morphology.
- T2-weighted images demonstrate the MS plaque as high signal.
- Post contrast T1-weighted images demonstrate enhancement of active MS plaques.
- FLAIR images improve MS plaque detection by suppressing CSF signal near the spinal cord.

**Treatment:** There is no specific treatment for MS.
- Corticosteroids and other drugs, however, are used to treat the symptoms.
- Physical therapy may help to postpone or prevent specific disabilities.

**Prognosis:**  The course of the multiple sclerosis disease process is varied and unpredictable.

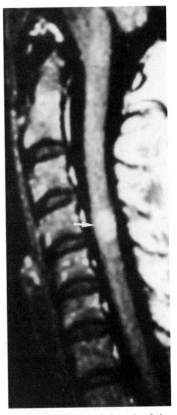

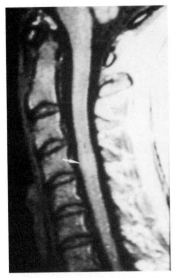

**FIGURE 1.  Multiple Sclerosis of the Spinal Cord.**  Noncontrast T1-weighted sagittal image shows an area of subtle increased signal intensity *(arrow)* of the spinal cord at the level of C4–C5.

**FIGURE 2.  Multiple Sclerosis of the Spinal Cord.**  Post contrast (gadolinium) T1-weighted sagittal image demonstrates a contrast-enhanced lesion *(arrow)* of the spinal cord at the level of C4–C5. This is consistent with an active MS plaque.

# SPINE
## TUMOR

## Spinal Ependymoma

**Description:** A spinal ependymoma is the most common tumor of the spinal cord. They are benign, slow growing, and arise from the ependymal cells lining the central canal or from ependymal rests.

**Etiology:** These tumors develop from ependymal cells lining the central canal or from ependymal rests.

**Epidemiology:** Males are slightly more affected than females. The peak incidence is in the fourth and fifth decade of life. The majority of all spinal ependymomas occur in the lumbosacral region.

**Signs and Symptoms:** Patients most commonly present with pain. Some patients may complain of leg weakness and sphincter dysfunction.

**Imaging Characteristics:** MRI is the imaging modality of choice for the diagnosis of spinal ependymoma.

### MRI
- Hypointense to isointense to the spinal cord on T1-weighted images.
- T2-weighted images produce a bright signal in the CSF and obscure the high signal of the tumor.
- Post contrast T1-weighted image shows a homogeneous, well-circumscribed, high-signal tumor.

**Treatment:** Complete surgical resection.

**Prognosis:** A complete resection of the tumor usually results in a cure.

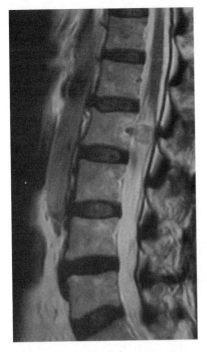

**FIGURE 1. Spinal Ependymoma.** T2-weighted sagittal MR image demonstrates a 1.3-cm round mass with intermediate signal in the conus medullaris at the level of L2.

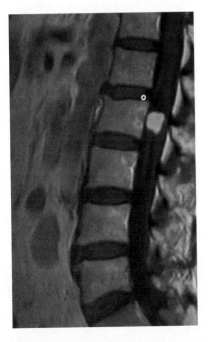

**FIGURE 2. Spinal Ependymoma.** Post contrast T1-weighted sagittal MR image demonstrates a round enhancing mass of the conus medullaris at the level of L2 consistent with an ependymoma.

# SPINAL HEMANGIOMA

**Description:** A vertebral hemangioma is the most common benign lesion incidentally found. Hemangiomas are slow-growing vascular tumors that generally do not cause symptoms. These lesions rarely result in compression or expansion of the vertebral body with subsequent cord compression.

**Etiology:** Unknown.

**Epidemiology:** Vertebral hemangiomas are the most common benign lesion of the spine and are present in more than 10 percent of all patients. Females are more affected than males by a ratio of 2:1. These lesions are most commonly located in the thoracic spine.

**Signs and Symptoms:** Nonspecific, these lesions are incidentally found.

## Imaging Characteristics:

### CT
- Bony striations associated with course, thickened trabeculae giving a "corduroy" appearance.
- Appear as low attenuation (hypodense) area

### MRI
- T1-weighted images appear hyperintense because of the presences of fat or hemorrhage.
- T2-weighted images appear hyperintense.

**Treatment:** Symptomatic treatment.

**Prognosis:** Excellent; hemangioma is a benign tumor.

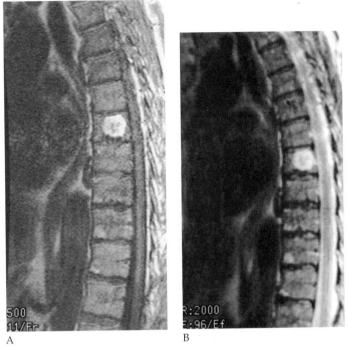

A                                    B

**FIGURE 1.  Spinal Hemangioma.**  T1-weighted (A) and T2-weighted (B) sagittal MR images demonstrate high signal intense, round lesion of the T-7 vertebral body consistent with hemangioma.

# SPINAL MENINGIOMA

**Description:** Spinal meningiomas are benign and account for approximately 25 percent of all intradural tumors. They are characteristically hard, slow growing, and usually highly vascular.

**Etiology:** Meningiomas of the spine are believed to arise from the arachnoid cells located near the dorsal nerve root ganglia.

**Epidemiology:** Meningiomas of the spine occur much less frequently than intracranial meningiomas. Spinal meningiomas usually present after the fourth decade of life and occur more commonly in females than males. They are found most commonly in the thoracic region (80 percent), followed by the cervical region (17 percent), and least often in the lumbar region (3 percent).

**Signs and Symptoms:** Patient presents with pain associated with compression of the spinal cord and adjacent nerve roots. Sensory and motor dysfunctions such as weakness, bowel and bladder dysfunction, and paresthesias may be present.

**Imaging Characteristics:** MRI is the imaging modality of choice for the diagnosis of spinal meningioma.

### CT
- Shows calcified meningiomas.
- CT myelography may demonstrate a blockage by an intradural/extramedullary mass.

### MRI
- T1-weighted images are typically isointense to the spinal cord.
- T2-weighted images may present with either low signal or high signal intensity.
- Contrast enhanced T1-weighted images show a homogeneous enhancing high signal intensity mass.

**Treatment:** Complete surgical removal.

**Prognosis:** Good; this is a benign tumor.

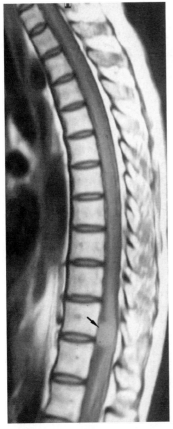

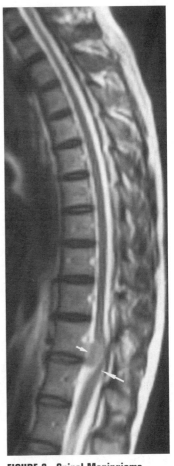

**FIGURE 1. Spinal Meningioma.**
T1-weighted sagittal image shows a round isointense mass *(arrow)* at the level of T6-T7.

**FIGURE 2. Spinal Meningioma.**
T2-weighted sagittal image shows a slightly high signal intensity mass *(short arrow)* at the level of T6-T7 displacing the cord *(long arrow)* posteriorly.

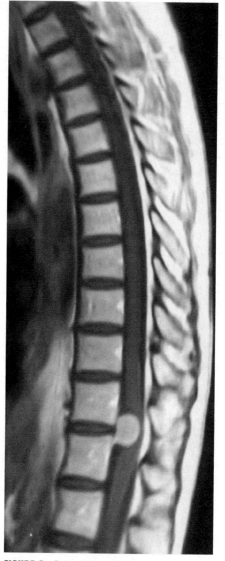

**FIGURE 3. Spinal Meningioma.** Post contrast
T1-weighted sagittal image shows intense
homogeneous enhancement of the mass at
the level of T6-T7.

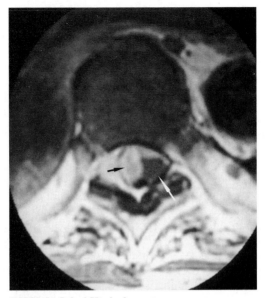

**FIGURE 4. Spinal Meningioma.** Post contrast
T1-weighted axial image shows a contrast enhancing
extramedullary mass in the right side of the spinal
canal *(short arrow)* at T6-T7, with displacement of
the cord *(long arrow)* to the left.

# METASTATIC DISEASE TO THE SPINE

**Description:** Metastatic tumors involving the bony vertebrae of the spine. These tumors are commonly a devastating complication of disseminated cancer.

**Etiology:** Metastatic spread of a cancer from a primary tumor. Metastases to the spine occur primarily as the result of hematogenous spread.

**Epidemiology:** Any malignant tumor can involve the vertebral spine; however breast carcinoma and lung carcinoma are the most common. Approximately 20 to 35 percent of all cancer patients develop symptoms associated with metastasis to the vertebral spine. Approximately 5 percent of affected patients develop symptoms related to spinal cord compression caused by the collapse of one or more vertebrae or by epidural tumor spread. The thoracic (70 percent) and lumbar (20 percent) regions are most commonly affected with 10 percent involving the cervical regions. There is a propensity for colon carcinoma to spread to the lumbosacral spine and breast and for lung carcinoma to metastasis to the thoracic spine.

**Signs and Symptoms:** Patient with known cancer history presents with back pain and possible loss of sensory and motor function. Suspected spinal cord compression requires emergent neurosurgical evaluation.

**Imaging Characteristics:** Plain x-rays and nuclear medicine bone scan, CT, and MRI are useful imaging modalities.

## CT
- CT is good for the evaluation of bone destruction.
- Shows osteolytic or osteoblastic bony metastatic lesion.

## MRI
- MRI is excellent for the evaluation of spinal cord compression.
- T1-weighted images appear with low signal intensity in the affected bony vertebrae.
- T2-weighted images appear with variable signal intensity in the affected bony vertebrae.
- Shows extension of the tumor into the spinal canal and spinal cord compression.

**Treatment:** Radiation therapy or surgery depending on the type of tumor. Spinal cord compression requires emergent radiation therapy or neurosurgery to prevent permanent paralysis.

**Prognosis:** A poor prognosis is expected for metastatic cancer.

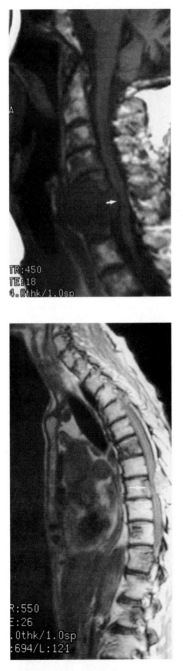

**FIGURE 1. Spinal Metastasis.**
T1-weighted sagittal image shows a large low signal intensity lesion involving the C5-C6 vertebral bodies with encroachment of the anterior spinal canal and compression of the spinal cord *(arrow)*.

**FIGURE 2. Spinal Metastasis.**
T1-weighted image shows low signal intensity lesions of multiple vertebrae. There is marked compression of the spinal cord at the level of T8 *(arrow)*.

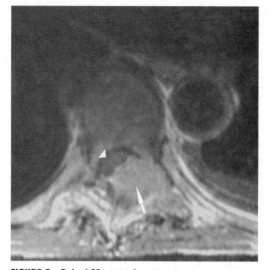

**FIGURE 3. Spinal Metastasis.** T1-weighted axial
image shows a high signal intensity mass *(arrow)*
encroaching on the spinal canal and compressing the
spinal cord *(arrowhead)*.

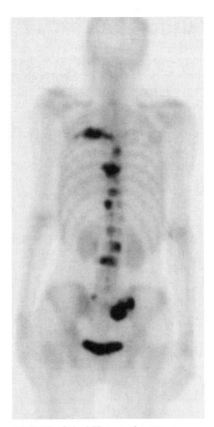

**FIGURE 4. Spinal Metastasis.** Whole-body bone scan shows multiple areas of increased uptake involving the thoracic and lumbar spine as well as the left pelvis and right upper ribs.

# VERTEBRAL OSTEOMYELITIS

**Description:** Osteomyelitis is an inflammation of the bone caused by an infecting organism. It may be localized or spread through the bone to involve the marrow, cortex, periosteum, and soft tissue surrounding the affected area. Vertebral osteomyelitis usually occurs as a result of disk space infection; however osteomyelitis may occur through hematogenous dissemination directly to the vertebral body. Pyogenic infections to the disk space are usually caused by a blood-borne pathogen from the lung or urinary tract. These pathogens get lodged in the region of the end-plate of the bone and destroys the disk space and the adjacent vertebral bodies.

**Etiology:** The majority (90 percent) of all bone and joint infections is caused by the Staphylococcus aureus microorganism and may occur following trauma or surgery. Other common infection-causing microorganisms include *Escherichia coli* and *Proteus*.

**Epidemiology:** Osteomyelitis can occur in any location and patients at any age. Patients that are particularly vulnerable include those who are diabetic, steroid users who are immunosuppressed, those patients on hemodialysis, and drug addicts, particularly heroin addicts.

**Signs and Symptoms:** Patient presents with fever, malaise, pain, and swelling over the affected area.

**Imaging Characteristics:** MRI is the preferred imaging modality. A gallium scan or indium-111–labeled leukocyte scan can also be helpful.

## MRI
- T1-weighted images show low signal intensity.
- T2-weighted images show high signal intensity.
- Post contrast, fat-suppressed, T1-weighted images show enhancement in bone as a result of abscess formation and juxtacortical soft tissue enhancement.

**Treatment:** Antibiotic treatment is required. Severe cases may also need surgery.

**Prognosis:** Generally good, with early diagnosis and effective treatment.

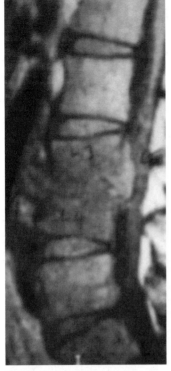

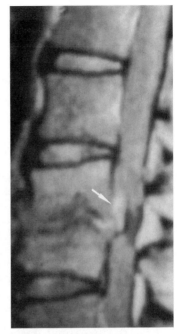

**FIGURE 1. Disk Space Infection (Vertebral Osteomyelitis).** T1-weighted sagittal image shows loss of normal L3-L4 disk. There is diffuse low marrow signal intensity of the L3-L4 vertebral bodies.

**FIGURE 2. Disk Space Infection (Vertebral Osteomyelitis).** Post contrast T1-weighted sagittal image shows a contrast enhancing mass *(arrow)* along the posterior aspect of L3-L4 disk consistent with an epidural abscess.

# SPINE
## TRAUMA

## BURST FRACTURE

**Description:** A vertically oriented fracture of the vertebral body with lateral dispersion of the fracture fragments, usually with associated fractures in the posterior elements of the vertebra (e.g., lamina and/or spinous process).

**Etiology:** Usually the result of a flexion or axial loading traumatic force, causing a flexion-compression injury.

**Epidemiology:** Most commonly occurs between 16- and 25 years of age. Males are more affected than females.

**Signs and Symptoms:** Patient presents with low back pain, possibly extending down the buttocks and backs of legs. Neurologic deficits, such as numbness and/or tingling in the lower extremities, leg weakness, or paralysis may be present.

**Imaging Characteristics:** CT is the imaging modality to demonstrate bony anatomy, while MRI is better for showing soft tissue structures.

### CT
- Fractures of vertebral body.
- Fractures of the pedicles and lamina.
- Shows displaced fracture fragments that may compromise the spinal canal.

### MRI
- Excellent modality to evaluate the status of the spinal canal and spinal cord.
- May show cord hemorrhage.
- May show compromise of the spinal canal and compression of the spinal cord.
- May show associated ligamentous injury or herniated disk.

**Treatment:** Surgical stabilization of the damaged bone or vertebra via fusing or metallic bracing may be required.

**Prognosis:** Mixed and varied, dependent upon the degree of damage and neurological involvement of spinal nerve roots and spinal cord.

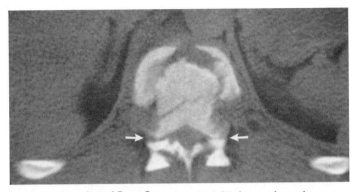

**FIGURE 1. Comminuted Burst Fracture.** Axial CT shows a burst fracture of T-12 with displacement of the fracture fragments resulting in compromise of the spinal canal. Note the fractures of the bilateral pedicles and associated small paraspinal hematoma (*arrows*).

# C1 Fracture

**Description:** Three primary types of fractures have been identified involving the C1 vertebrae: (1) the posterior arch fracture, which usually occurs at the junction of the posterior arch and the lateral mass; (2) the lateral mass fracture, which usually occurs unilaterally with the fracture line passing either through the articular surface or just anterior and posterior to the lateral mass on one side; and (3) the burst fracture (Jefferson fracture), which is characterized by four fractures, two in the anterior arch and two in the posterior arch. This fracture may present as a stable nondisplaced fracture with no encroachment on the spinal cord or as a displaced fracture with varying degrees of encroachment on the spinal cord. A displaced fracture with encroachment on the spinal cord may cause morbidity (i.e., paralysis), or death.

**Etiology:** Fractures to C1 occur as a result of axial loading to the top of the head (e.g., swimming and diving related accidents). The degree of injury depends on the magnitude of the axial loading and whether the spine is in flexion, neutral or an extension position.

**Epidemiology:** Trauma to the spine occurs more commonly in the cervical region than in any other area of the spine.

**Signs and Symptoms:** The patient may present with pain or possible neurologic deficit.

**Imaging Characteristics:** CT is the modality of choice for the diagnosis of a C1 fracture.

## CT
- Noncontrast study with bone window setting shows fracture of the C1 vertebrae.
- May demonstrate other related bony or soft tissue injuries to the upper cervical region.

## MRI
- Useful in evaluating the spinal cord and other soft tissue structures of the spine.

**Treatment:** Most fractures of the C1 vertebrae can be treated with immobilization (e.g., rigid cervical orthosis or a halo vest).

**Prognosis:** Depends on the degree of injury and other associated injuries.

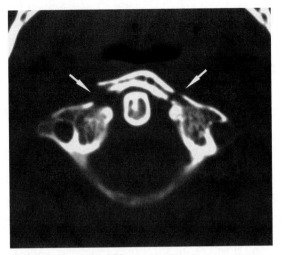

**FIGURE 1. Fracture of C1.** Axial CT of C1 demonstrate fractures of the anterior arch *(arrows)*.

# VERTEBRAL COMPRESSION FRACTURE

**Description:** Compression fractures of the lumbar spine occur as a result of a combination of flexion and axial loading (compression) of the vertebrae.

**Etiology:** This fracture can occur as a result of trauma, metastatic disease to the spine or osteoporosis.

**Epidemiology:** Compression fractures are common in the aging and geriatric patient with osteoporosis.

**Signs and Symptoms:** Patient presents with back pain and possible neurological deficit.

**Imaging Characteristics:** CT is the imaging modality to demonstrate bony anatomy, while MRI is better for showing soft tissue structures and spinal cord.

## CT
- Shows fracture of vertebral body.
- Shows fractures of the pedicles and lamina.
- Shows displaced fracture fragments that may compromise the spinal canal.
- Thin-section multiplanar images are very useful.

## MRI
- Excellent modality to evaluate the status of the spinal canal and spinal cord.
- May show cord hemorrhage.
- May show compromise of the spinal canal and compression of the spinal cord.
- May show associated ligamentous injury or herniated disk.

**Treatment:** These injuries are usually stable because the bony posterior elements and longitudinal ligaments are intact.

**Prognosis:** Depends on the extent of the injury and status of the spinal canal and cord.

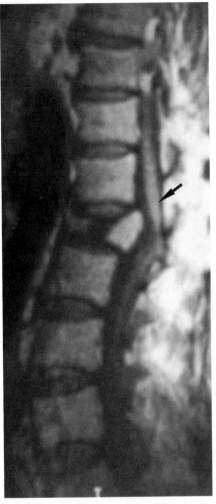

**FIGURE 1.  Compression Fracture L1.**
T1-weighted sagittal image shows severe
compression fracture of the L1 body. There is
a posterior displacement (retrolisthesis) with
displacement and compression *(arrow)* of the
spinal cord (conus).

# Spinal Cord Hematoma

**Description:** A spinal cord hematoma is a collection of blood in the spinal cord, most commonly caused by trauma.

**Etiology:** Most spinal cord hematomas occur as a result of trauma to the spinal cord, ligamentous structures, and/or bony vertebra. Other associated causes may include an acute herniated disk or hemorrhage from an arteriovenous malformation.

**Epidemiology:** Trauma to the spinal column occurs at an incidence of approximately 2 to 5 per 100,000 population. Many of these injuries are a result of motor vehicle accidents. Less-frequent causes include falls, diving accidents, and sports and recreational injuries. Adolescents and young adults, especially males, are more commonly affected.

**Signs and Symptoms:** Depending on the level and extent of the injury, the patient may present with motor and sensory dysfunction.

**Imaging Characteristics:** Plain x-rays of the spine should be done first. CT is good for the evaluation of bony structures, whereas MRI is excellent for the evaluation of soft tissue and spinal cord. Extrinsic changes include disk herniation and ligamentous injury. Intrinsic changes include edema and hemorrhage.

## MRI

1. Acute stage (several hours to 3 days).
   - Slightly low signal on T1-weighted images.
   - Marked low signal with high signal on surrounding edema on T2-weighted images.

2. Subacute stage (3 days to 3 weeks).
   - High signal on T1-weighted images.
   - High signal with low signal clot on T2-weighted images.

3. Chronic stage (3 weeks to months).
   - High signal on T1-weighted images.
   - High signal with low signal rim on T2-weighted images.
   - Gradient echo images appear with low signal intensity.

**Treatment / Prognosis:** Presence of a spinal cord hematoma indicates a poor prognosis. Permanent neurologic deficit is most likely.

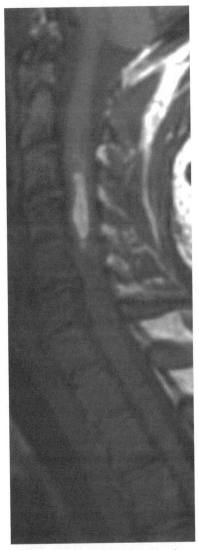

**FIGURE 1. Hemorrhagic Contusion of the Spinal Cord.** T1-weighted sagittal MRI of the cervical spine shows high signal intensity within the spinal cord at the C3-C5 level consistent with a hemorrhage. There is also swelling of the cord from C2-C4.

# FRACTURE/DISLOCATION: (C6–C7)

**Description:** Spinal subluxation is the partial dislocation of the spinal vertebrae. Facet dislocations may be either stable (unilateral) or unstable (bilateral) in more severe cases. A subluxation of the spinal vertebrae is associated with either a partial or complete disruption of the posterior longitudinal ligament and the anterior longitudinal ligament. In many cases, this may be associated with a fracture of either facet at the level of the dislocation.

**Etiology:** Traumatic conditions that result in hyperextension or hyperflexion and rotation of the cervical spine.

**Epidemiology:** Cervical spine subluxation is associated with hyperextension and hyperflexion related traumatic injuries to the cervical column.

**Signs and Symptoms:** Patient presents with pain and possible neurologic deficit.

**Imaging Characteristics:** Plain films should be done first for screening.

## CT
- Useful in identifying bony injury (fracture) extent of fracture, status of posterior elements, and spinal canal.
- Spiral CT (single or multidetector) with thin sections (1 to 3 mm) sagittal and coronal reformatted.

## MRI
- Excellent for the evaluation of the spinal cord and other soft tissue injuries.

**Treatment:** Reduction of the fracture/dislocation.

**Prognosis:** Depends on the extent of the trauma and status of the spinal cord. The presence of cord hemorrhage is generally considered to be a poor prognosis.

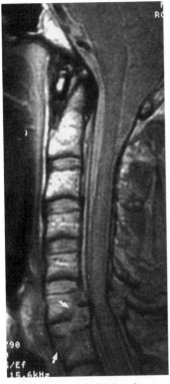

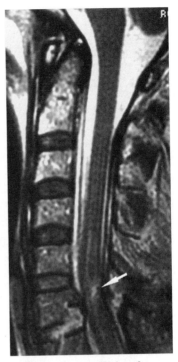

**FIGURE 1. Fracture/Dislocation of C6–C7.** T1-weighted sagittal image of the cervical spine demonstrates a fracture of the posterior inferior aspect of the C6 and anterior superior aspect of C7 vertebral body *(arrows)*. There is an anterior displacement of C6 vertebral body over C7. There is a displaced C6 fracture fragment into the anterior spinal canal causing spinal cord compression.

**FIGURE 2. Fracture/Dislocation of C6–C7 with Cord Edema.** T2-weighted sagittal image shows a focal increased signal intensity *(arrow)* of the spinal cord at the C6 level representing cord edema. There is no hemorrhage.

# ODONTOID FRACTURE

**Description:** Fractures of the odontoid process or dens are classified into three types. A type I fracture, rarely seen, is an avulsion of the tip of the dens. Type II is the most common and consists of a fracture through the base of the dens. Type III fractures extend through the upper body of the C-2 vertebrae.

**Etiology:** Fractures of the dens usually result from extreme flexion of the head.

**Epidemiology:** Trauma to the spine occurs more commonly in the cervical region than in any other area of the spine.

**Signs and Symptoms:** Patient may present with pain or a varying degree of neurologic deficit.

**Imaging Characteristics:** Spiral CT is the modality of choice for the diagnosis of an odontoid fracture.

## CT
- Noncontrast study with sagittal and coronal reformatted bone window images show fracture of the dens.
- May demonstrate other related bony or soft-tissue injuries to the upper cervical spine.

## MRI
- Useful in evaluating the spinal cord and other soft tissue structures.

**Treatment:** Depending on the type of fracture, immobilization with a halo vest and possible bony fusion may be successful.

**Prognosis:** Depends on the type of fracture and status of the spinal cord.

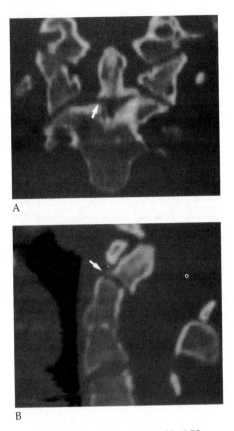

A

B

**FIGURE 1. Fracture of the Odontoid of C2.**
Coronal (A) and sagittal (B) reformatted
images demonstrate a transverse fracture
(*arrows*) of the base of the odontoid of C2
(type II fracture). There is some posterior
displacement of the odontoid.

# SPINE

## VASCULAR DISEASE

# Spinal Cord Ischemia/Infarction

**Description:** Ischemia and infarction of the spinal cord is the decrease or absence of blood to the spinal cord.

**Etiology:** Most result from atherosclerosis, hypertension, thoracoabdominal aortic aneurysm, sickle cell anemia, caisson disease, diabetes, meningitis, and spinal trauma.

**Epidemiology:** The lower thoracic cord and conus are most commonly involved.

**Signs and Symptoms:** The patient presents with diminished bowel and bladder function, loss of perineal sensation, and reduced sensory and motor function of the lower extremities.

**Imaging Characteristics:** MRI is the imaging modality of choice for the diagnosis of spinal cord ischemia or infarction.

### MRI
- T1-weighted images may show an enlargement of the spinal cord.
- T2-weighted images show high signal intensity in the cord.
- FLAIR images are very helpful by suppressing the CSF signal.

**Treatment:** Treatment is usually symptomatic.

**Prognosis:** Depends on the extent and severity of the infarct.

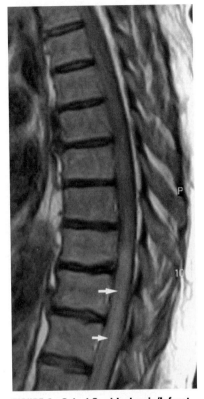

**FIGURE 1. Spinal Cord Ischemia/Infarct.**
FLAIR sagittal image of the thoracic
spine shows an enlargement with
diffuse increased signal intensity
(*arrows*) of the distal thoracic spinal
cord.

# PART III

# Head and Neck

# CONGENITAL

## BRACHIAL CLEFT CYST

**Description:** Brachial cleft cysts are congenital anomalies and usually arise from the second brachial arch during embryologic development. During clinical presentation the cystic mass appears in the anteriolateral portion of the neck around the angle of the mandible.

**Etiology:** Congenital anomaly.

**Epidemiology:** Bimodal age distribution. The first occurrence is at birth with the second peak seen in young adults. About 10 percent are bilateral in location.

**Signs and Symptoms:** This cystic mass is usually painless.

**Imaging Characteristics:** Shows well-defined round cystic mass posteriolateral to the submandibular gland. There is no contrast enhancement.

### CT
• Shows cyst as low density.

### MRI
• T1-weighted image is hypointense.
• T2-weighted image is hyperintense.

**Treatment:** Complete surgical resection.

**Prognosis:** Good.

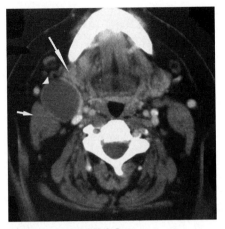

**FIGURE 1. Brachial Cleft Cyst.** Postcontrast axial CT demonstrates an approximate 3×3-cm well-defined, round, benign-appearing cystic mass *(arrowhead)* along the anterior medial aspect of the right sternocleidomastoid muscle *(short arrow)* and posteriolateral to the right submandibular gland *(long arrow)* consistent with a second brachial cleft cyst.

# TUMOR

## GLOMUS (CAROTID BODY) TUMOR (PARAGANGLIOMA)

**Description:** A glomus tumor or paraganglioma is a benign, slow-growing, hypervascular lesion. They are named according to their anatomic location such as *glomus vagale* (most common) when in the carotid space above the carotid bifurcation. Others, such as *glomus jugulare*, are associated with the jugular foramen; and *glomus tympanicum* is associated with the middle ear.

**Etiology:** This is a benign tumor arising from the neural crest paraganglion cells of the extracranial head and neck.

**Epidemiology:** These lesions may be multiple in 5 percent of the patients; almost 30 percent of patients have a familial history of the disease.

**Signs and Symptoms:** Depends on the location of the tumor.

**Imaging Characteristics:**

### CT
- Contrast-enhanced study demonstrates an enhancing, well-circumscribed, soft tissue mass.

### MRI
- T1-weighted images show mixed signal intensity mass with multiple signal (flow) voids.
- Paragangliomas produce a high signal on T2-weighted images.
- Postcontrast T1-weighted images of the tumor are hyperintense with signal (flow) voids giving it a salt-and-pepper appearance.

**Treatment:** May require surgery, radiation therapy, or both.

**Prognosis:** Good; this is a benign tumor.

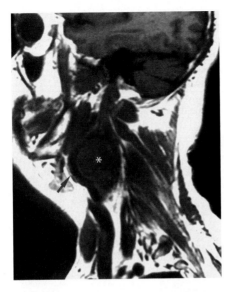

**FIGURE 1. Carotid Body Tumor (Glomus Tumor).** T1-weighted left parasagittal image shows an intermediate signal mass *(asterisk)* of the upper neck at the carotid bifurcation. The external carotid artery *(arrow)* is displaced anteriorly.

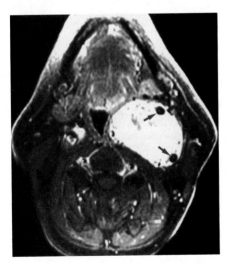

**FIGURE 2. Carotid Body Tumor (Glomus Tumor).** Postcontrast T1-weighted axial image shows a large markedly enhancing mass of the upper neck splaying the internal and external *(arrows)* carotids above the common carotid artery bifurcation.

# Cavernous Hemangioma (Orbital)

**Description:**  Cavernous hemangiomas of the orbit are the most common benign orbital tumor in adults.

**Etiology:**  These vascular malformations are composed of large, dilated, endothelium-lined vascular channels covered by a fibrous capsule.

**Epidemiology:**  These slow progressive tumors usually occur in patients between the second and fourth decades of life and are slightly more common in females. These tumors are usually located intraconal, but extraconal cavernous hemangiomas are possible.

**Signs and Symptoms:**  Patients present with painless proptosis (bulging eyes).

## Imaging Characteristics:

### CT
- Appear as well-defined, high-density, smooth-margined, homogeneous, rounded, ovoid (egg-shaped), or lobulated mass with marked contrast enhancement.

### MRI
- T1-weighted images demonstrate an isointense to hypointense well-circumscribed mass.
- The tumor appears hyperintense to fat on T2-weighted images.
- Postcontrast T1-weighted images show marked enhancement.

**Treatment:**  Surgical resection of these encapsulated benign tumors is the recommended treatment of choice.

**Prognosis:**  Surgical resection produces a high cure rate.

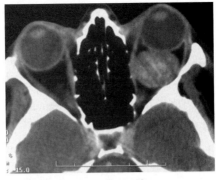

**FIGURE 1.  Cavernous Hemangioma.**
Noncontrast CT showing smoothly marginated,
high-density, round, contrast-enhancing
intraconal mass of the left orbit displacing the
left globe anteriorly.

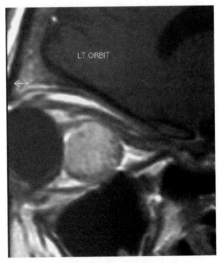

**FIGURE 2.  Cavernous Hemangioma.** Sagittal
T1-weighted MR shows round slightly
hyperintense retrobular mass displacing
optic nerve superiorly.

# Parotid Gland Tumor (Benign Adenoma)

**Description:** The salivary glands can be divided into major and minor types. The major salivary glands include the parotid, submandibular, and sublingual glands. The parotid gland is the largest salivary gland and forms the majority of salivary neoplasms. The minor salivary glands are comprised of hundreds of smaller glands distributed throughout the mucosa and aerodigestive tract.

**Etiology:** Radiation is suspected to be a cause of both benign and malignant lesions.

**Epidemiology:** The average age to acquire a parotid gland tumor is between the fourth and fifth decade of life. Greater than 80 percent of parotid gland tumors are benign mixed tumors (pleomorphic adenomas). The tendency for malignant tumors increases in the submandibular, sublingual and the minor salivary glands.

**Signs and Symptoms:** Benign tumors are usually palpable, discrete, and mobile. Malignant tumors commonly present as a palpable lump or mass. Pain, rapid expansion, poor mobility or facial nerve weakness are additional symptoms associated with malignancy.

**Imaging Characteristics:** Mass effect may displace surrounding anatomy.

## CT
- Shows round mass with density similar to that of muscle against fatty background of the normal parotid gland.
- Demonstrates mild to moderate contrast enhancement.

## MRI
- Lesions are best identified on T1-weighted images amid the bright signal of parotid fat.
- Benign tumors are very bright on T2-weighted images.
- Malignant tumors are hypointense on T2-weighted images.

**Treatment:** Surgical removal for benign tumors. For malignant parotid gland tumors, complete surgical resection with radiation therapy is indicated.

**Prognosis:** Good; 80 percent of parotid gland tumors are benign. For those that are malignant, the patient outcome depends on the staging of the cancer and early detection and treatment. The overall 10-year survival rates for stages I, II, and III are approximately 90 percent, 65 percent, and 22 percent, respectively.

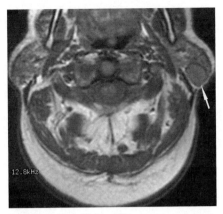

**FIGURE 1. Parotid Gland Tumor.** T1-weighted axial MRI of the parotid gland demonstrates a well-defined, round, low signal intensity mass *(arrow)* in the posterior aspect of the superficial lobe of the left parotid gland.

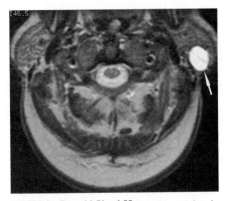

**FIGURE 2. Parotid Gland Mass.** T2-weighted axial MRI of the parotid gland demonstrates a well-defined, high signal intensity mass *(arrow)* of the posterior aspect of the superficial lobe of the left parotid gland consistent with a pleomorphic adenoma.

# SUBMANDIBULAR SALIVARY GLAND ABSCESS

**Description:** Submandibular salivary gland abscesses are mucus-filled retention cysts derived from obstructed or traumatized salivary ducts.

**Etiology:** May be caused by a stone in the submandibular duct, or in the gland itself. Inflammation of the submandibular lymph nodes may arise secondary to a dental abscess, or an infective lesion of the tongue, floor of the mouth, mandible, cheek or neighboring skin.

**Epidemiology:** Unknown.

**Signs and Symptoms:** Abscesses are associated with skin thickening, edema of the fat, and gas in more than 50 percent of cases. They are also associated with pain and tenderness in the area of the affected gland.

**Imaging Characteristics:**

## CT
- Low-density cystic mass.
- May show variable contrast enhancement.
- May show calcified submandibular duct stone.

## MRI
- Hypointense on T1-weighted images.
- Hyperintense on T2-weighted images.

**Treatment:** Submandibular swelling may be treated with antibiotics. Surgical intervention may be required in select cases.

**Prognosis:** Good with early diagnosis and treatment.

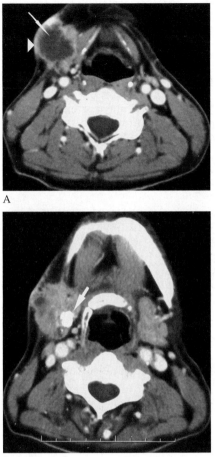

A

B

**FIGURE 1. Abscess of the Submandibular Salivary Gland.** (A) Postcontrast CT shows enlarged right submandibular gland with central low density *(small arrow)* and irregular peripheral contrast enhancement *(arrowhead).* Postcontrast axial CT (B) image demonstrates a calcified stone *(arrow)* in the right submandibular gland. These findings are consistent with an abscess of the right submandibular gland secondary to an obstruction from a stone (calculus).

# SINUS

## MUCOCELE

**Description:** Mucoceles arise as a complication associated with sinusitis. They are the most common expansive lesion involving the paranasal sinuses.

**Etiology:** Mucoceles tend to occur as a consequence of a long-standing obstruction of the paranasal sinuses.

**Epidemiology:** Mucoceles most commonly affect the frontal sinus. Maxillary and ethmoid sinuses combined comprise approximately a third of all mucoceles. The sphenoid sinus is rarely involved.

**Signs and Symptoms:** Because mucoceles are noninfected lesions, they typically present clinically with symptoms associated with mass effect.

**Imaging Characteristics:**

**CT**
- Complete opacification and expansion of the sinus with thinned walls.
- There may be bony erosion of the sinus wall.

**MRI**
- Most appear low signal intensity on T1-weighted images and high signal intensity on T2-weighted images.
- Some may appear dilated but aerated (inspissated) and are hypointense on both T1- and T2-weighed images.

**Treatment:** Surgery drainage of the sinus cavity.

**Prognosis:** Good with early diagnosis and treatment.

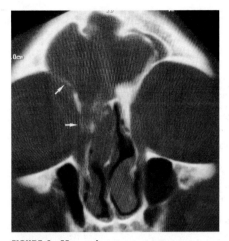

**FIGURE 1. Mucocele.** Coronal CT image demonstrate complete opacification and expansion of right frontal and ethmoid sinuses. Note that there is thinning and bone erosion of the lateral walls of the frontal and ethmoid sinuses *(arrows).*

# SINUSITIS

**Description:** Sinusitis is an acute or chronic inflammation of the paranasal sinuses.

**Etiology:** Bacterial, viral, or fungal infections may cause sinusitis.

**Epidemiology:** All ages can be affected. Males and females are equally affected.

**Signs and Symptoms:** Nasal congestion, a feel of pressure building around the orbital area and associated headache, malaise, and fever are common indicators of sinusitis. Patients may also experience sore throat or an occasional cough.

**Imaging Characteristics:** Coronal CT is the best imaging plane for the evaluation of sinus diseases.

## CT
- Examination of the sinuses reveals mucosal thickening, opacification, or air-fluid levels in one or more of the paranasal sinuses.
- CT also shows obliteration of ostiomeatal complex (common drainage area for frontal, anterior ethmoid and maxillary sinuses).

**Treatment:** Steam inhalation may aid the patient in providing comfort and encourage drainage. Antibiotics, analgesics, antihistamines may also be used to treat sinusitis. Preventative measures include allergy testing, avoiding cigarette smoking, and avoiding extreme changes in temperature.

**Prognosis:** A good prognosis should be expected.

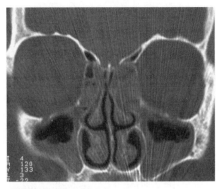

**FIGURE 1. Sinusitis.** Coronal CT of the sinuses shows moderate thickening of the bilateral maxillary sinuses and marked opacification of the bilateral ethmoid sinuses. There is obliteration of the bilateral ostiomeatal complex.

# TRAUMA

## INTRAOCULAR FOREIGN BODY

**Description:** An intraocular foreign body is one of several injuries that may result from ocular trauma. An intraocular foreign body occurs as a result of an object penetrating and remaining in the orbit.

Ocular trauma may result from any of the following: (1) globe disruption; (2) lens dislocation; (3) intraocular foreign body; or (4) hemorrhage. In the case of an intraocular foreign body, an object has penetrated the orbit.

**Etiology:** Injuries may occur at home, in the workplace, during recreation or as auto accidents. Many injuries are occupationally related, such as, metal workers and construction workers. In some cases, injuries may result from BB guns or other small projectile objects.

**Epidemiology:** Males are more commonly affected than females. Although all ages can be affected, the median age is in the second and third decades of life.

**Signs and Symptoms:** The patient usually states "something has hit them in the eye." Pain and discomfort are the initial symptoms.

### Imaging Characteristics:

### CT
- Shows opaque foreign bodies in the orbit.
- Shows bony fractures in the orbital area.
- Shows hemorrhage in the orbital area.

### MRI
- The presence of an intraocular metallic foreign body is a contraindication to performing an MRI due to the possibility of an ocular injury occurring from movement of a ferromagnetic substance.

**Treatment:** Surgery is usually required.

**Prognosis:** Good, if the foreign body is outside the globe.

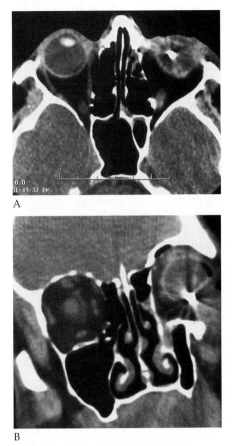

A

B

**FIGURE 1. Intraocular Foreign Body.** Axial
(A) and coronal (B) noncontrast CT of the
orbits demonstrates a small metallic foreign
body within the inferior aspect of the left
globe. There is no evidence of hemorrhage.
Note the metallic artifacts from the foreign
body.

# TRIPOD FRACTURE

**Description:**  The tripod fracture is the most common facial fracture. It is comprised of three fractures involving the zygomatic arch, orbital floor or rim, and the maxillary process.

**Etiology:**  This injury results from a blunt force blow to the area of the zygoma.

**Epidemiology:**  It may happen to anyone who experiences a blunt force blow to the area of the zygoma.

**Signs and Symptoms:**  Pain and swelling in the "cheek" area of the face, bruising, facial disfigurement.

**Imaging Characteristics:**

**CT**
- CT is the preferred modality.
- Axial and coronal images are needed for the evaluation of the full extent of the injury.
- Shows fractures of the zygomatic arch, posteriolateral wall of the maxillary sinus and the orbital floor and rim.
- Opacification of maxillary sinus, secondary to blood.

**Treatment:**  Surgery is usually required.

**Prognosis:**  Depends on the extent of the injury, and other associated injuries (e.g., brain hemorrhage).

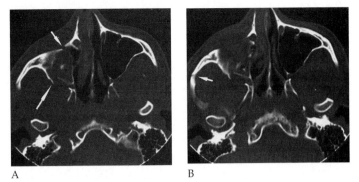

A                              B

**FIGURE 1. Tripod Fracture.** Axial CT of facial bones (A) demonstrates fractures of the anterior *(small arrow)* and posteriolateral *(large arrow)* walls of the right maxillary sinus. In (B), there is also a fracture of the right zygomatic arch *(arrow)*.

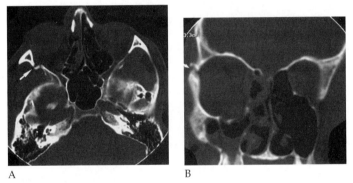

A                              B

**FIGURE 2. Tripod Fracture.** Axial and coronal CT of the facial bones shows a fracture of the lateral wall of the right orbit (A, *arrow*), as well as diastasis (separation) of the right frontozygomatic suture (B, *arrow*).

# PART IV

# Chest and Mediastinum

# LUNGS

## BRONCHOGENIC CARCINOMA

**Description:**  Lung cancer is any of the various primary malignant neoplasms that may appear in the lung. Lung cancer is the leading cause of death from cancer in both men and women.

**Etiology:**  The exact cause of lung cancer is unknown, however inhalation of carcinogens is known to be a predisposing cause. Cigarette smoking is by far the most important risk factor for the development of carcinoma of the lung.

**Epidemiology:**  Lung cancer is rarely found in individuals under the age of 40 years. The incidence rate rises rapidly after the age of 50 years, with 60 years being the average age of occurrence. The majority of cases appear between 50 and 75 years of age. The occurrence ratio is 2:1 male to female.

**Signs and Symptoms:**  Patients may present with any combination of the following: cough, hemoptysis, dyspnea, pneumonia, chest pain, shoulder pain, arm pain, weight loss, bone pain, hoarseness, headaches, seizures, or swelling of face or neck.

**Imaging Characteristics:**  Chest x-ray is usually done first although there is some debate regarding spiral CT for screening of lung cancer.

### CT
- Appears as a mass with irregular speculated margins.
- There may be central necrosis with large tumors.
- CT is good for staging of lung cancer (i.e. metastatic mediastinal lymph nodes, liver, and adrenal metastasis).

**Treatment:**  Surgery, radiation therapy, and chemotherapy may be used depending on the staging and type of cancer.

**Prognosis:**  Depending on the stage of the cancer, the 5-year survival rate varies from just greater than 50 percent for patients with stage I disease to approximately 15 percent for those with stage III disease.

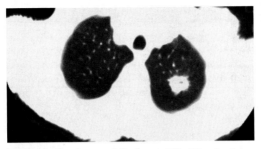

**FIGURE 1. Carcinoma of the Lung.** CT of the chest
with lung windows demonstrates a round mass with
irregular speculated margins in the left upper lobe.

# BULLOUS EMPHYSEMA

**Description:** Emphysema is one of the many chronic obstructive pulmonary diseases affecting the lungs. Emphysema involves the destruction of the alveolar wall. This reduces the surface area for gas exchange and allows the collection of free air on inhalation to accumulate in the lung tissue.

**Etiology:** Cigarette smoking is the most common cause associated with the development of this disease. In a rare form of emphysema, a congenital deficiency in the production of the protein antitrypsin is associated with the development of emphysema in young adults.

**Epidemiology:** It is estimated that more than 60,000 deaths per year are related to emphysema. It usually occurs after the fourth decade of life and is more commonly seen in males.

**Signs and Symptoms:** Patients will typically present with dyspnea, chronic cough, weight loss, malaise, barrel chest, pursed lip breathing, minimal wheezing, and the use of accessory muscles to assist respiration.

### Imaging Characteristics:

**CT**
- Hyperinflation of the lungs.
- Lucent, hypodense (dark) areas of the lung surrounded by normal lung parenchyma. These hypodense sharply demarcated areas measuring 1 cm or greater in diameter are commonly referred to as blebs or bullae and represent the collection of "free air" trapped within the lung during the breathing (inhalation) process and unable to be exhaled.

**Treatment:** Smoking cessation, administration of oxygen, and eating a well balanced diet are common methods of treatment. Lung reduction surgery may be indicated in select cases.

**Prognosis:** Depends on the extent of the disease, however, an improved prognosis is expected if the patient quits smoking, eats a balanced diet, and uses supplemental oxygen.

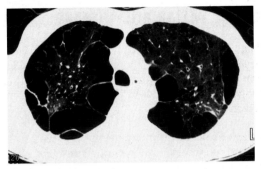

**FIGURE 1. Bullous Emphysema.** CT of the chest shows multiple bullae of the bilateral upper lobes in the subpleural location.

# PULMONARY METASTATIC DISEASE

**Description:** The lung is frequently the site of metastatic disease from primary cancers outside the lung. Metastatic spread to the lung is usually considered to be incurable. A solitary pulmonary lesion may represent a metastasis process or a new primary lung cancer.

**Etiology:** The lungs are the most frequent site of metastatic spread. Metastatic spread is accomplished through the blood circulation or lymphatic system.

**Epidemiology:** Carcinoma of the kidney, breast, pancreas, colon, and uterus are the most likely to metastasize to the lungs.

**Signs and Symptoms:** The most common symptom is a cough. Other related symptoms include hemoptysis, wheezing, fever, dyspnea, and chest pain.

**Imaging Characteristics:** CT is the modality of choice for imaging pulmonary metastatic disease.

## CT
- Typically shows multiple bilateral lung masses that are noncalcified.
- May also show mediastinal lymphadenopathy.

**Treatment:** Surgical resection when possible. Radiation therapy may be used when tumors are inoperable, and chemotherapy for palliative use.

**Prognosis:** Poor.

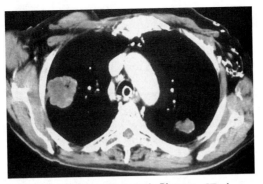

**FIGURE 1. Pulmonary Metastatic Disease.** CT of the chest with mediastinal windows demonstrating bilateral upper lobe masses with areas of low density representing necrosis.

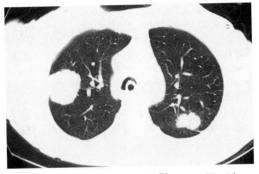

**FIGURE 2. Pulmonary Metastatic Disease.** CT with lung window showing bilateral upper lobe masses with slightly irregular margins consistent with metastatic lesions.

# PULMONARY EMBOLI

**Description:** A pulmonary embolus (PE) is an obstruction of the pulmonary artery or one of its branches by an embolus.

**Etiology:** Generally results from dislodged thrombi originating in the leg veins. Risk factors include long-term immobility, chronic pulmonary disease, congestive heart failure, recent surgery, advanced age, pregnancy, fractures or surgery to the lower extremities, burns, obesity, malignancy and use of oral contraceptives.

**Epidemiology:** This is the most common pulmonary complication in hospitalized patients. The incidence rate of new cases is between 600,000 and 700,000 annually with 100,000 to 200,000 deaths. Men and women are equally affected. Advancing age increases risk of developing pulmonary emboli.

**Signs and Symptoms:** Chest pain, shortness of breath, hemoptysis (coughing of blood), and swelling of legs.

**Imaging Characteristics:** Spiral CT pulmonary angiography (CTPA) is the best noninvasive test for diagnosing PE and is gradually replacing the ventilation/perfusion (V/Q) lung scan. CT is reliable in diagnosing emboli in larger central pulmonary arteries but may miss small emboli in smaller subsegmental peripheral pulmonary arteries which may not be clinically significant.

## CT

- IV contrast study demonstrates a hypodense plug-like structure within the pulmonary artery.
- Filling defects in the pulmonary arteries.
- Obstruction of the pulmonary arteries.
- Combined CTPA and CT venography (CTV) may show filing defects in the iliac and femoral veins.

**Treatment:** Depending on the size and location of the emboli and the patient's condition, the patient may be treated with oxygen as needed, IV heparin, warfarin, and/or thrombolytic therapy.

**Prognosis:** Good with early diagnosis and treatment. Large saddle emboli can be fatal.

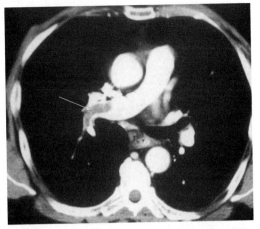

**FIGURE 1. Pulmonary Emboli.** CTPA shows large filling defect (clot) in the right main pulmonary artery *(arrow)* extending into the lower lobe pulmonary arteries.

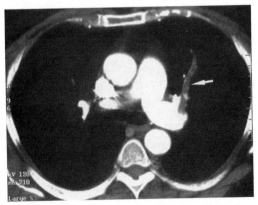

**FIGURE 2. Pulmonary Emboli.** CTPA shows linear filling defect representing a clot in the left upper lobe pulmonary artery *(arrow)*.

# MEDIASTINUM

## HODGKIN'S DISEASE

**Description:** Hodgkin's disease is a primary neoplastic malignancy of the lymphatic system. It is characterized by painless enlargement of the lymph nodes, spleen, and other lymphatic tissues. Histologic evaluation is made by identifying the classic Reed-Sternberg cell.

**Etiology:** The exact cause is unknown, however, the Epstein-Barr virus is a possible etiologic agent.

**Epidemiology:** Hodgkin's disease accounts for less than 1 percent of all malignancies and for 14 percent of all malignant lymphomas. There is a bimodal age distribution. The first peak occurs between 15 and 35 years of age and the second between 55 and 75 years. This malignancy occurs more often in males than in females.

**Signs and Symptoms:** Patients may experience painless, palpable lymph node(s), dry cough, weight loss (greater than 10 percent), fever, and night sweats.

**Imaging Characteristics:** CT is the preferred modality to diagnosis mediastinal and retroperitoneal lymphadenopathy.

### CT
- Enlarged mediastinal lymph nodes.
- Enlarged retroperitoneal and mesenteric lymph nodes.
- Enlarged spleen and liver.

**Treatment:** Radiation therapy may be used to administer a tumoricidal dose, chemotherapy is used typically with a combined multidrug regimen and surgery is usually used for biopsy purposes only or for splenectomy.

**Prognosis:** Generally good with early diagnosis and treatment.

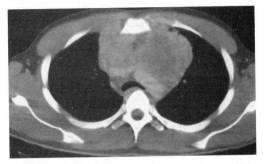

**FIGURE 1. Hodgkin's Disease.** Contrast-enhanced CT shows a very large anterior mediastinal mass displacing the aortic arch posteriorly and compressing the trachea. This mediastinal mass in this young patient is consistent with lymphoma or Hodgkin's disease.

# AORTA

## AORTIC DISSECTION

**Description:** An aortic dissection occurs when blood enters into the wall of the artery dissecting between the layers and creating a cavity or false lumen in the vessel wall. Dissecting aneurysms are classified into two types according to the Stanford classification scale. Dissecting aneurysms involving the ascending aorta are classified as Type A. Those involving only the descending aorta are Type B.

**Etiology:** Most likely results from a tearing of the wall of the artery.

**Epidemiology:** The peak incidence occurs in the 6th and 7th decades of life. Males are more commonly affected than females. Approximately 60 percent of dissecting aneurysms are Type A and 40 percent are Type B. The most common predisposing condition is hypertension. Other predisposing factors include Marfan syndrome, coarctation, bicuspid aortic valve, aortitis, and pregnancy. Aortic dissection may be iatrogenic and result at the site of an aortic cannulation, bypass grafting, cross-clamping, or during a catheterization procedure.

**Signs and Symptoms:** Patients may present with pain in the chest or abdomen. Approximately 15 to 20 percent of patients present asymptomatic.

**Imaging Characteristics:** CT with IV contrast is the best (readily available and faster) imaging modality for the evaluation of aortic dissection.

### CT
- Precontrast images may show enlarged aorta, intimal flap, and intimal calcification.
- Precontrast images show the thrombosed false lumen with a higher attenuation value.
- Precontrast images show pericardial, mediastinal, and/or pleural hemorrhage as secondary to rupture.
- Postcontrast images show contrast-filled true and false lumens separated by the intimal flap.
- Postcontrast images show a delayed enhancement of the false lumen.

- Postcontrast images show compression of the true lumen by the thrombosed false lumen.
- Postcontrast images show ischemia/infarction or organs supplied by vessels branching from the false lumen.

## MRI
- Good for the evaluation of an aortic dissection.
- MRI/MRA (magnetic resonance angiography) offers multiplanar imaging and no need for IV contrast.
- Shows same findings as CT.

**Treatment:** Depends on the type (Stanford classification) of dissecting aneurysm. Type A dissections, those involving the ascending aorta, usually require surgery. Type B dissecting aneurysms are usually managed medically to control hypertension.

**Prognosis:** Good with Type B dissection. If untreated, Type A dissection has a high mortality and may result in cardiac tamponade.

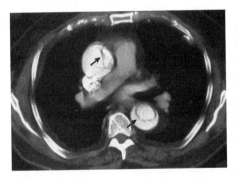

**FIGURE 1. Type A Dissecting Aneurysm.** Axial CT with IV contrast demonstrates a Type A aortic dissecting aneurysm involving both the ascending and descending thoracic aorta showing a double lumen separated by the intimal flap (*arrow*).

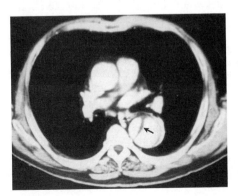

**FIGURE 2. Type B Dissecting Aneurysm.** Axial CT with IV contrast shows a Type B dissecting aneurysm involving the descending thoracic aorta with two lumens (true and false) separated by an intimal flap (*arrow*).

# Aortic Tear

**Description:** An aortic tear involves a traumatic tearing or laceration of the aorta.

**Etiology:** The majority of these cases are associated with high-speed motor vehicle (deceleration) accidents. Others may occur as a result of falls, crushing injuries, or blast related (compression) injuries.

**Epidemiology:** More than 90 percent of aortic tears occur at the aortic isthmus (just distal to the origin of the left subclavian artery). This is the site where the ligamentum arteriosum attaches to the aortic arch and the pulmonary artery.

**Signs and Symptoms:** Many patients do not demonstrate any visible external signs of chest trauma. However, as a result of head trauma, a great number of these patients present with altered mental status. In patients with a history involving a rapid deceleration, the possibility of an aortic injury is suspected.

## Imaging Characteristics:

### CT
- A mediastinal hematoma occurs in association with the tear.
- Loss of normal contour of the aorta at the site of the tear.
- Extravasation of contrast.
- Periaortic hematoma.
- Small aortic tears may be difficult to visualize.

**Treatment:** Emergency surgical intervention.

**Prognosis:** 80 to 90 percent of all patients with aortic laceration/tear die at the scene of the accident or are dead on arrival at the hospital. For the 10 to 20 percent of patients who arrive at the hospital alive, a rapid diagnosis and surgical repair can produce survival rates. However, other injuries related to the initial traumatic event may complicate the patient's recovery.

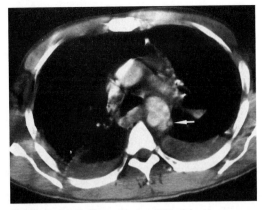

**FIGURE 1. Aortic Tear.** Contrast CT of the chest shows contour irregularity with extravasation *(arrow)* of contrast in the thoracic aorta. There are small bilateral pleural effusions.

# BREAST

## BREAST IMPLANT LEAKAGE

**Description:** Silicone gel-filled breast implants were first used in patients in the early 1960s. Initially, silicone exposure was thought to represent a health risk to women with breast implants. To date, however, scientific evidence supporting an association between silicone gel-filled breast implants and classic autoimmune disease are unclear. Virtually all silicone gel-filled breast implants "bleed" small amounts of silicone fluid through the intact implant shell. This is not to be confused with larger amounts of "leakage" of silicone gel caused by a rupture in the structural integrity of the implant shell.

**Etiology:** Causes for implant leakage (i.e., bleeding or rupture) are unclear, but possibilities include upper body exercise and activity, submuscular placement, trauma, mammography, and weak implant wall design.

**Epidemiology:** In 1999, there were an estimated 2 million women with breast implants in the United States. The absolute rupture rate of implants in the general population of all implant patients has yet to be measured. Reported implant rupture rates for patients seen for known or suspected problems have ranged anywhere from 23 percent to 92 percent.

**Signs and Symptoms:** Patients with breast implant silicone-gel leakage may be asymptomatic.

**Imaging Characteristics:** MRI is useful in the evaluation of the breast implant. The fluid in breast implants appears with similar signal intensities as cerebrospinal fluid.

### MRI

- Good for evaluating the integrity of the breast implant (e.g., intact, herniation, partially or complete rupture, intracapsular and extracapsular).
- With extracapsular rupture MRI shows collection of silicone outside the implant lumen.
- Intracapsular rupture demonstrates presence of multiple curvilinear low signal intensity lines commonly referred to as the linguine sign and is seen within the high-signal silicone gel.

**Treatment:**  Surgical removal of ruptured implants, and evacuation of silicone or polyurethane when possible.

**Prognosis:**  Postsurgical prognosis should be good, barring unforeseen complications.

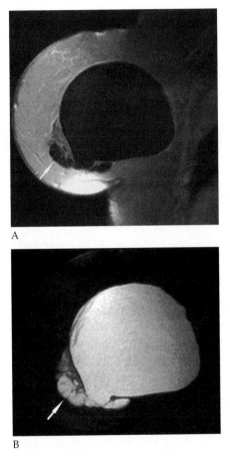

A

B

**FIGURE 1.  Rupture of Breast Implant.** T1-weighted (A) and T2-weighted (B) MR images of the breast show collections of silicone *(arrows)* outside the implant lumen that are diagnostic of extracapsular rupture.

# TRAUMA

## PNEUMOTHORAX

**Description:** A pneumothorax is a collection of air within the pleural cavity.

**Etiology:** Primarily results from traumatic blunt injury to the chest.

**Epidemiology:** A pneumothorax occurs in up to 40 percent of patients experiencing blunt trauma to the chest. It may be associated with or without rib fractures. A laceration of the visceral pleura from a rib fracture is seen in approximately 70 percent of cases. Young males in their second to fourth decade are more commonly affected.

**Signs and Symptoms:** The patient presents with chest pain and dyspnea.

**Characteristics:** Plain x-ray is the primary choice for detecting and evaluating a pneumothorax. CT is useful in evaluating difficult cases such as a small pneumothorax in the supine patient.

### CT
- A collection of fluid and air is seen within the pleural cavity.
- Rib fractures may be seen penetrating into the chest.
- Lung contusions or lacerations may be seen.
- Associated abdominal injuries may be seen.

**Treatment:** A thoracostomy (chest) tube may be inserted to reexpand the lung. Surgical intervention may be required in severe cases.

**Prognosis:** Depends on the extent of the pneumothorax and other associated injuries. A good recovery should be expected.

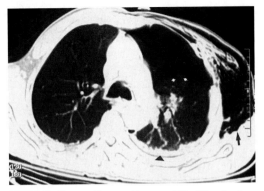

**FIGURE 1. Pneumothorax.** Contrast CT of the chest shows large left pneumothorax with air outlining the visceral pleura *(short arrows)*. There is minimal hemothorax *(arrowhead)*. There is a large subcutaneous emphysema *(long arrows)* of the left chest wall.

# PART V

## Abdomen

# LIVER

## CAVERNOUS HEMANGIOMA

**Description:** Cavernous hemangiomas are the most benign hepatic tumors. Found as either single or multiple tumors, they are usually small measuring 1 to 2 cm in diameter. These tumors are mostly silent with only a small percentage being symptomatic.

**Etiology:** Composed primarily of large vascular channels.

**Epidemiology:** Occurs in all age groups. Is more common in females than males. The incidence rate is approximately 1 to 2 percent in the normal adult population and up to 20 percent at autopsy.

**Signs and Symptoms:** Usually an incidental finding on large symptomatic tumors; upper abdominal pain is experienced.

### Imaging Characteristics:

#### CT
- Noncontrast studies appear hypodense.
- Early peripheral contrast enhancement whereas the central portion of the lesion remains low density. Sequential scan over a period of time demonstrates progressive contrast filling of the lesion; central, low density, progressively becoming smaller.

#### MRI
- T1-weighted images appear hypointense.
- T2-weighted images appear hyperintense.
- T1-weighted contrast enhanced images appear hyperintense with increasing signal over 15 to 30 minutes following injection.

**Treatment:** Surgical intervention is usually not required unless the tumor is large and symptomatic.

**Prognosis:** Good; these are benign tumors.

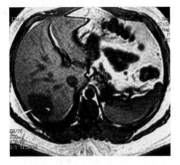

**FIGURE 1. Cavernous Hemangioma.**
T1-weighted MRI of the liver
shows round, low signal intensity
mass (*arrow*) in the posterior
segment of the right lobe of the
liver.

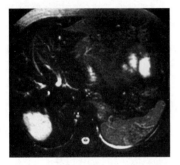

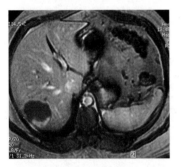

**FIGURE 2. Cavernous Hemangioma.**
T2-weighted MRI of the liver
shows this lesion to be very bright
(high signal intensity).

**FIGURE 3. Cavernous Hemangioma.**
Early postcontrast gradient echo
MRI of the liver shows peripheral
enhancement of the mass lesion.

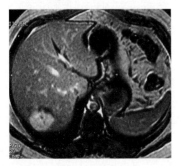

**FIGURE 4. Cavernous Hemangioma.**
Delayed postcontrast gradient echo
MRI of the liver shows contrast
filling of this lesion.

# FATTY INFILTRATION OF THE LIVER

**Description:** Fatty infiltration of the liver is the result of excessive depositions of triglycerides and other fats in the liver cells.

**Etiology:** This condition appears in association with a variety of disorders such as obesity, malnutrition, chemotherapy, alcohol abuse, steroid use, parenteral nutrition, Cushing syndrome, and radiation hepatitis. In the United States, the most common cause is related to alcoholism.

**Epidemiology:** In the United States, this disorder is commonly associated with the overuse of alcohol.

**Signs and Symptoms:** Fatty liver is usually "silent" but may be associated with hepatomegaly and abdominal pain in the right upper quadrant.

**Imaging Characteristics:** CT is the modality of choice for diagnosing fatty infiltration of the liver.

## CT
- Fatty infiltrates may be focal or diffusely distributed within the liver.
- Fatty infiltrates demonstrate a lower (hypodense) attenuation in appearance in comparison to the spleen on noncontrast studies.

## MRI
- T1- and T2- weighted images may demonstrate an increase in signal when compared to normal liver parenchyma.
- The STIR sequence suppresses the signal from fat when compared to above pulse sequences.

**Treatment:** Supportive and consists of correcting the underlying condition or eliminating its cause (e.g., alcohol) and focusing on proper nutrition.

**Prognosis:** Depends on the underlying condition or etiology.

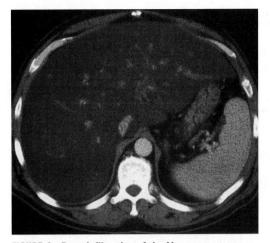

**FIGURE 1. Fatty Infiltration of the Liver.** CT of the abdomen with IV contrast shows mildly enlarged liver. There is diffuse low attenuation of the liver, when compared to the spleen, which is consistent with fatty infiltration. Note the contrast opacified hepatic and portal veins against the low-density background of the liver appear bright.

# HEPATIC CYSTS

**Description:**  Simple hepatic cysts found in the liver.

**Etiology:**  Liver cysts are thought to be congenital.

**Epidemiology:**  These lesions are commonly found in roughly 5 to 10 percent of the general population.

**Signs and Symptoms:**  Hepatic cysts are asymptomatic. They are usually an incidental finding.

**Imaging Characteristics:**  Hepatic cysts may appear as single or multiple cysts.

## CT
- Appear as a homogeneous, well-defined, round or oval-shaped, thin-walled lesion.
- The cysts have a near-water attenuation value that should not enhance with IV contrast.

## MRI
- T1-weighted images appear hypointense.
- T2-weighted images appear hyperintense.
- T1-weighted contrast enhanced images will show no enhancement.

**Treatment:**  There is no treatment required for hepatic cysts.

**Prognosis:**  Because these lesions are incidental findings and are asymptomatic with no known side effects, the prognosis for these cysts are good.

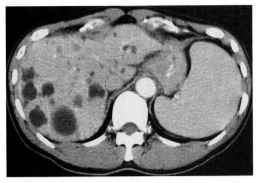

**FIGURE 1. Liver Cysts.** CT of the abdomen with IV contrast demonstrates multiple low-density lesions in the liver. These lesions have a near-water CT attenuation value and smooth margins consistent with cysts.

# HEPATIC METASTASES

**Description:** Metastatic spread of cancer to the liver involves the deposit of cancer cells into the liver parenchyma. Metastatic liver disease occurs more frequently than primary liver malignancies.

**Etiology:** Liver metastases can originate from essentially any primary malignancy, but most commonly spreads from the gastrointestinal tract, especially the colon. Other cancers that frequently metastasize to the liver include gastric, pancreatic, breast, lung, ovary, kidney, and carcinoid tumors of the intestinal tract which tend to occur in the terminal ileum or appendix.

**Epidemiology:** The liver is the second most common site (lungs are the most commonly affected) for metastatic spread of cancer.

**Signs and Symptoms:** May present with abdominal pain, jaundice and possibly a palpable mass.

**Imaging Characteristics:** Contrast-enhanced CT is the modality of choice. MRI is useful when CT is inconclusive.

## CT
- Well-defined low-attenuation (hypodense) solid masses when compared to the liver parenchyma on noncontrast studies.
- Some tumors may show contrast enhancement.
- Calcifications or hemorrhage may be seen in the metastatic masses on noncontrast CT.

## MRI
- T1-weighted images show hypointense metastatic lesion.
- T2-weighted images may show hypointense, isointense, or hyperintense metastatic lesions.
- Gadolinium enhanced T1-weighted images show hypointense lesions.

**Treatment:** Depends on the cancer staging. Chemotherapy may be used singularly or in combination with conservative surgical resection when metastasis is localized to three or fewer segments.

**Prognosis:** Poor; depends on the stage of the primary cancer.

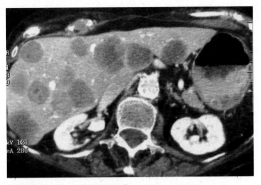

**FIGURE 1. Liver Metastasis.** Contrast-enhanced CT of the abdomen demonstrates multiple round, hypodense lesions throughout the liver, consistent with liver metastasis.

# HEPATOMA

**Description:** A hepatoma, also known as hepatocellular carcinoma (HCC) is the most common primary malignant liver tumor. It accounts for approximately 75 percent of liver cancers.

**Etiology:** Risk factors associated with hepatitis B infection include, alcohol-induced cirrhosis, aflatoxin (a mold that grows on rice and peanuts) contaminated food, anabolic steroids, thorotrast (thorium dioxide, a contrast medium formerly used in liver radiography), and immunosuppressive agents.

**Epidemiology:** There are anywhere from one to five new cases each year. The average age of detection is between the fifth and sixth decades of life. Males are affected more than females at a ratio of 3:1. There is a very high incidence rate associated with individuals who are from China, Southeast Asia, western and southern Africa, Taiwan, and Hong Kong.

**Signs and Symptoms:** Patient may present with a palpable mass, abdominal pain in the right upper quadrant (RUQ), hepatomegaly, weight loss, nausea, and vomiting, and may be a known cirrhosis patient.

### Imaging Characteristics:

#### CT
• Appears hypodense on noncontrast study.
• CT with IV contrast show variable enhancement.

#### MRI
• T1-weighted images appear hypointense.
• T2-weighted images appear hyperintense.
• T1-weighted contrast enhanced images show variable enhancement.

**Treatment:** Surgical intervention to remove the tumor prolongs life and may improve the patient's quality of life. The presence of cirrhosis reduces the patient's prognosis. Radiation therapy and chemotherapy are used to provide some degree of palliation.

**Prognosis:** Surgical resection of the tumor is the treatment of choice. Unfortunately, 85 to 90 percent of the cases are not surgical resectable.

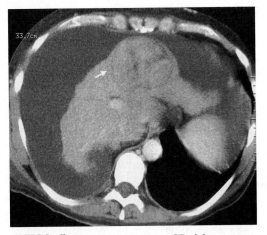

**FIGURE 1.  Hepatoma.**  Postcontrast CT of the upper abdomen shows a small irregular liver with massive ascites consistent with cirrhosis. There is an 8×6-cm, round, solid mass (*arrow*) in the anterior aspect of the dome of the right lobe of the liver consistent with a hepatoma.

# HEPATOBILIARY

## CHOLEDOCHAL CYST

**Description:** A choledochal cyst is a focal dilatation of the bile duct.

**Etiology:** A choledochal cyst is considered to be a congenital anomaly of the biliary tree.

**Epidemiology:** More commonly seen in females than males. Patients may be clinically symptomatic before 10 years of age.

**Signs and Symptoms:** Although not seen in all patients, the classic clinical triad of symptoms includes pain, jaundice, and a palpable abdominal mass in the upper right quadrant.

**Imaging Characteristics:** A cystic dilatation of the extrahepatic bile, with or without dilatation of the intrahepatic bile duct.

### CT
- Demonstrates a cystic mass in the porta hepatis that appears with an approximate density of water.

### MRI
- Low signal from within the cyst is seen on T1-weighted images.
- High signal from within the cyst is seen on T2-weighted images.
- MR cholangiopancreatography (MRCP) is the best noninvasive test for the diagnosis of choledochal cyst.
- MRCP shows localized dilation of the common bile duct.

**Treatment:** Surgical resection is often performed because of the risk of malignancy associated with this disorder.

**Prognosis:** If the obstruction is not corrected, infections and chronic liver disease can develop. In the case of a cancerous tumor, complete resection and therapy produce a 30 to 40 percent 5-year survival rate.

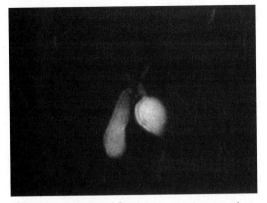

**FIGURE 1. Choledochal Cyst.** MRCP in the coronal plane shows a fusiform dilatation of the common bile duct. This is consistent with a type I choledochal cyst.

# CHOLEDOCHOLITHIASIS

**Description:** Choledocholithiasis is a calculi or stone in the common bile duct. These calculi usually form in the gallbladder and move into the common bile duct.

**Etiology:** Stones consisting primarily of cholesterol are primarily developed in the gallbladder and enter into the common bile duct.

**Epidemiology:** Approximately 10 to 15 percent of patients with cholecystitis have stones in the common bile duct. The incidence rate increases with age and is seen more frequently in females.

**Signs and Symptoms:** The patient is asymptomatic when there is no obstruction. Abdominal pain in the epigastric region, nausea and vomiting, with a loss of appetite, fever, and jaundice usually indicate an obstruction of the common bile duct. Other signs could include pancreatitis and a palpable gallbladder.

## Imaging Characteristics:

### CT
- Stones with a high attenuation (hyperdense) may be seen without IV contrast.

### MRI
- MR cholangiopancreatography (MRCP) is the best noninvasive study for the diagnoses.
- MRCP demonstrates the stone as hypointense defect in the common bile duct (CBD).

**Treatment:** Endoscopic retrograde cholangiopancreatography (ERCP) with sphincterotomy and stone removal in most cases. Surgical removal is rarely needed.

**Prognosis:** Good with early diagnosis and treatment. The patient may experience complications secondary to obstruction of the CBD such as jaundice, cholangitis, and pancreatitis.

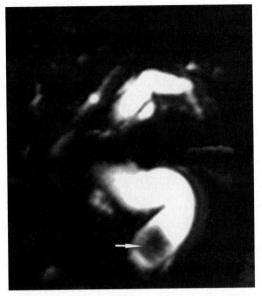

**FIGURE 1. Choledocholithiasis.** MRCP in the coronal plane shows low signal intensity (*arrow*) defect within the distal common bile duct consistent with a stone.

# PANCREATIC ADENOCARCINOMA

**Description:** Pancreatic adenocarcinoma is the second most common visceral malignancy and the fifth leading cause of cancer mortality.

**Etiology:** Although there is no known cause, there is evidence that suggests there is a link to inhalation or absorption of certain carcinogens found in cigarettes, foods high in fat and protein, food additives, industrial chemicals (betanaphthalene, benzidine, and urea). Additional possible predisposing factors are chronic pancreatitis, diabetes mellitus, and chronic alcohol abuse.

**Epidemiology:** There are approximately 28,000 new cases diagnosed annually with about 26,000 deaths. It occurs most commonly between the fourth and seventh decade of life. The majority of these tumors are located in the head of the pancreas.

**Signs and Symptoms:** Patients usually present with weight loss, abdominal pain, and jaundice. Jaundice is caused by an obstruction of the bile ducts by the pancreatic tumor (head).

**Imaging Characteristics:** Contrast CT is the preferred imaging modality; MRI is used in difficult cases.

### CT and MRI
- Mass in the head of the pancreas (66 percent of patients).
- Dilated bile ducts, pancreatic duct secondary to obstruction of the distal common bile duct (CBD) by the tumor in the head of the pancreas.
- Invasion or encasement of adjacent vascular structures by pancreatic tumor.
- Liver metastasis.
- Enlarged metastatic lymph nodes.

**Treatment:** Although surgery offers the best hope for cure, roughly 80 percent of the patients at diagnosis are ineligible for curative treatment. Radiation therapy may be helpful. Chemotherapy has not proven to improve the patient's condition.

**Prognosis:** Poor. The average survival following pancreatic resection is approximately 17 months.

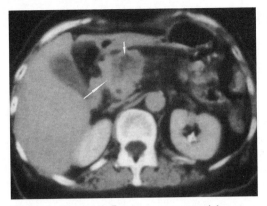

**FIGURE 1. Pancreatic Tumor.** Contrast CT of the abdomen shows large irregular mass of the head of the pancreas (*long arrow*) causing obstruction of the distal common bile duct. Note the central low-density area within the mass representing necrosis (*short arrow*).

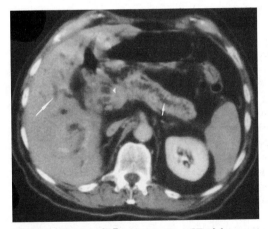

**FIGURE 2. Pancreatic Tumor.** Contrast CT of the abdomen shows dilated intrahepatic bile ducts (*long arrow*). There is also dilated pancreatic duct (*short arrow*) as well as common bile duct (*arrowhead*).

# PANCREATIC PSEUDOCYST

**Description:** Pancreatic pseudocysts are composed of a collection of cellular debris, old blood, and pancreatic fluid that has become encapsulated in a fibrous sac.

**Etiology:** Pseudocysts of the pancreas may occur as a result of pancreatic inflammation and trauma.

**Epidemiology:** Patients who recently experienced a bout of acute pancreatitis or trauma to the pancreas are potential candidates to develop pseudocyst.

**Signs and Symptoms:** Patients present with a palpable mass, abdominal pain, nausea and vomiting, loss of appetite, and jaundice.

## Imaging Characteristics:

### CT
- Appears as a well-defined, round, low-density, thick- or thin-walled capsule, and has a near-water attenuation value.

### MRI
- The pseudocyst appears with a low signal (hypointense) region on T1-weighted images and with a high signal on T2-weighted images.

**Treatment:** Pancreatic pseudocysts may resolve spontaneously. For those that do not resolve or that increase in size, drainage is usually required, either through a CT-guided catheter or surgical drainage.

**Prognosis:** Depends on complications associated with extent and severity of the pseudocyst and treatment. In the more serious cases, there can be a high morbidity and mortality rate.

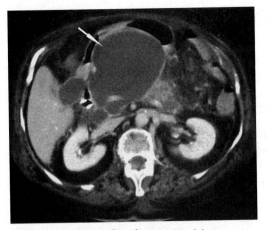

**FIGURE 1. Pancreatic Pseudocyst.** CT of the
abdomen with IV contrast demonstrates a large,
round, low-density mass (*arrow*) in the region of
the head of the pancreas with displacement of the
stomach and duodenum. This cystic mass has a near-
water CT attenuation value consistent with a cyst.

# PANCREATITIS

**Description:** Pancreatitis is an inflammation of the pancreas, and occurs in acute and chronic forms. The difference between the acute and chronic forms is based on the restoration of normal pancreatic function in the former and permanent residual damage in the latter.

**Etiology:** The most common cause of pancreatitis is alcoholism. Other causes include gallstones, trauma, pancreatic cancer, certain drugs, postendoscopic retrograde cholangiopancreatography (ERCP), and metabolic disorders (hypertriglyceridemia, hypercalcemia, renal failure).

**Epidemiology:** The incidence rate is between 10 and 20 per 100,000 populations. Acute pancreatitis can occur at any time; however, chronic pancreatitis tends to occur between 35 and 45 years of age and is usually linked with alcohol intake. Males and females are equally affected.

**Signs and Symptoms:** Patients may present with abdominal pain, nausea and vomiting, mild abdominal distention, fever, hypotension, mild jaundice, reduced or absent bowel sounds, umbilical discoloration (Cullen sign), and pleural effusion.

**Imaging Characteristics:** CT is the imaging modality of choice.

## CT
- Diffuse enlargement of the pancreas.
- Soft-tissue stranding of the peripancreatic fat and thickening of the fascia.
- Intrapancreatic and peripancreatic fluid collection.
- Pancreatic pseudocyst may be seen.
- Pancreatic calcification may be seen in chronic pancreatitis.

**Treatment:** Medical treatment is mostly symptomatic with the focus being to prevent and treat the complications. Pancreatic abscess and pseudocysts can be treated with CT-guided catheter drainage. Surgery may be necessary in some cases.

**Prognosis:** Depends on the underlying condition or etiology as well as the complications associated with pancreatitis.

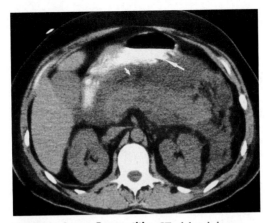

**FIGURE 1. Severe Pancreatitis.** CT of the abdomen without IV contrast demonstrates diffuse enlargement of the pancreas. Fluid collection is noted along the anterior aspect of the pancreas within the lesser sac (*short arrow*), with displacement of the barium-opacified stomach anteriorly (*long arrow*). Note the thickening of the renal fascia on the left kidney.

# GENITOURINARY

## AGENESIS OF THE KIDNEY

**Description:** Renal agenesis is the congenital absence of one of the kidneys.

**Etiology:** Renal agenesis is a congenital anomaly.

**Epidemiology:** Unilateral agenesis of the kidney occurs in approximately 1 of every 500 patients, and is more commonly found in males than females (3:1 ratio).

**Signs and Symptoms:** In many cases renal agenesis is an incidental finding.

### Imaging Characteristics:

### CT and MRI
- Absence of a kidney.
- Compensatory hypertrophy of existing kidney, renal nein, and adrenal gland.

**Treatment:** There is no treatment for this condition. Patient education and monitoring for preventative measures might be advised.

**Prognosis:** Depending on renal function, the patient may live a normal life.

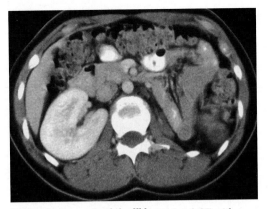

**FIGURE 1. Agenesis of the Kidney.** Axial CT with contrast shows an absence of the left kidney with compensatory hypertrophy of the right kidney.

# ANGIOMYOLIPOMA

**Description:** Angiomyolipomas are fairly common benign renal tumors composed of three components: (1) fat, (2) blood vessels, and (3) smooth muscles. *Hamartoma* is associated with a benign mass composed of disorganized tissues normally found in an organ, while *choristoma* implies a benign mass of disorganized tissues not normally found in an organ.

**Etiology:** A tumor composed of an overgrowth of mature cells and tissues normally present in the affected area (i.e., blood vessels, smooth muscle tissue, and fat).

**Epidemiology:** Angiomyolipomas are more commonly seen in females than in males, ranging from 40 to 60 years of age. Approximately 20 percent of all patients diagnosed with angiomyolipomas have multiple, bilateral masses, and are associated with tuberous sclerosis.

**Signs and Symptoms:** Patients present with abdominal pain, palpable mass, hemorrhage, and hematuria.

## Imaging Characteristics:

### CT
- The detection of the fat in this renal mass assists with confirming the diagnosis of angiomyolipoma.

### MRI
- T1- and T2-weighted images will appear with high signal (hyperintense).
- T1-weighted fat-suppression technique allows fat within the tumor to be distinguished from hemorrhage.

**Treatment:** Surgical intervention is required if life-threatening hemorrhaging occurs. Angioembolization can also be used.

**Prognosis:** Angiomyolipoma are benign tumors. Mortality is usually secondary to bleeding or hemorrhage of the tumor.

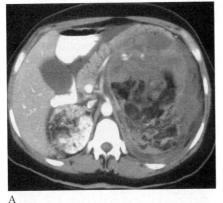

A

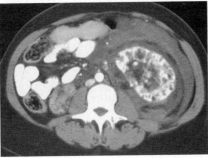

B

**FIGURE 1. Renal Angiomyolipoma.** CT abdomen with IV contrast demonstrates a large left perinephric hematoma (A and B) secondary to bleeding from the angiomyolipoma of the left kidney. Note the multiple fat-density tumors in both kidneys.

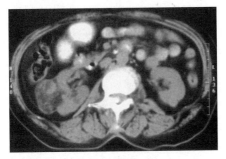

**FIGURE 2. Renal Angiomyolipoma.**
Noncontrast CT of the abdomen of another patient shows round mixed density mass in the lateral aspect of the right kidney. These are fat densities within the right renal mass consistent with an angiomyolipoma.

# HORSESHOE KIDNEY

**Description:** A horseshoe kidney is a congenital anomaly characterized by the fusion of the lower (90 percent) or upper (10 percent) poles of the kidney. This produces a horseshoe-shaped structure continuous across the midline and anterior to the great vessels.

**Etiology:** Horseshoe kidney is a congenital anomaly.

**Epidemiology:** This anomaly is considered to be common and is found in approximately 1 of every 500 patients.

**Signs and Symptoms:** This condition is usually asymptomatic but there can be complications such as ureteropelvic junction (UPJ) obstruction, infections, and stone formation.

## Imaging Characteristics:

### CT
- Demonstrates a horseshoe-shaped kidney fused more commonly at the lower pole (90 percent) of the time or at the upper pole (10 percent) of the time.

### MRI
- T1-weighted imaging is best used to visualize this anatomic renal anomaly.

**Treatment:** This congenital anomaly is usually seen as an incidental finding and requires no treatment.

**Prognosis:** Depending on renal function, the patient should live a normal life.

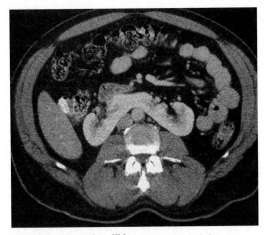

**FIGURE 1. Horseshoe Kidney.** CT of the abdomen with IV contrast demonstrates fusion of the lower pole of both kidneys seen crossing the midline anterior to the aorta and inferior vena cava.

# PERINEPHRIC HEMATOMA

**Description:** A perinephric hematoma is a collection of blood that is confined to Gerota fascia (i.e., perirenal fascia) and arises as a result of blunt or penetrating trauma to the kidney.

**Etiology:** Blunt or penetrating trauma to the abdominal area.

**Epidemiology:** Renal injuries occur in approximately 10 percent of trauma victims. Most renal injuries are associated with motor vehicle accidents. It is common for a hemorrhage to occur in the perinephrotic space following a renal biopsy.

**Signs and Symptoms:** Depending on the extent of the injury and time to treatment, patients may present with abdominal pain, an open wound, signs of internal bleeding with blood in the urine, increased heart rate, declining blood pressure, and hypovolemic shock, nausea and vomiting, decreased alertness, and moist, clammy skin.

**Imaging Characteristics:** Contrast-enhanced CT is the modality of choice for the evaluation of abdominal or renal trauma.

## CT
- Hyperdense in appearance on acute noncontrast studies.
- Hypodense area surrounding the contrast-enhanced kidney.
- Shows associated laceration of kidney.
- Follow-up CT for stable patient with conservative treatment to monitor resolution of hematoma.

**Treatment:** Surgical intervention may be required in emergent situations for the hemodynamically unstable patient. Conservative treatment for the stable patient may include bed rest, analgesics, and patient monitoring.

**Prognosis:** Depends on the extent of the injury, patient response to treatment, and any other associated injuries.

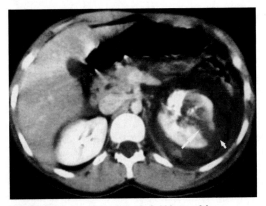

**FIGURE 1. Laceration of the Left kidney with Perinephric Hematoma.** CT of the abdomen with IV contrast shows low-density areas of the parenchyma of the left kidney consistent with deep (*long arrow*) grade 3 laceration and hematoma. There is also a hematoma (*short arrow*) surrounding the left kidney.

# Polycystic Kidney Disease

**Description:**  Adult polycystic kidney disease (PKD) is an inherited disorder characterized by multiple fluid-filled cysts of varying sizes. These cysts cause lobulated enlargements of the kidneys that result in cystic compression and progressive failure of the renal tissue.

**Etiology:**  Adult polycystic kidney disease is a hereditary (autosomal dominant) disorder.

**Epidemiology:**  Incidence rate is between 1 and 5 in 1000 population. Males and females are equally affected. PKD is usually diagnosed between the third and fourth decade of life. PKD accounts for 5 to 10 percent of patients with end-stage renal disease.

**Signs and Symptoms:**  Patients may present with hypertension, hematuria, palpable kidneys, hepatomegaly, abdominal pain, and flank pain. An association between PKD and the presence of cerebral berry aneurysms exists.

## Imaging Characteristics:

### CT
- Multiple hypodense or cystic masses involving one or both kidneys.
- Enlarged kidneys.

### MRI
- Enlarged kidneys with multiple cysts that have a low signal on T1-weighted images and a high signal on T2-weighted images.

**Treatment:**  PKD is incurable. Treatment is aimed at preserving renal parenchyma and preventing infectious complications. Managing hypertension helps prevent rapid deterioration in function. Progressive renal failure requires treatment such as dialysis or, rarely, kidney transplant.

**Prognosis:**  Slowly progressive, with a variable outcome. End-stage renal disease occurs in 70 percent of patients by age 65 years.

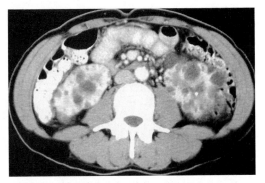

**FIGURE 1. Adult Polycystic Kidney Disease.** CT of the abdomen with IV contrast demonstrates enlarged bilateral kidneys with numerous cysts of varying sizes.

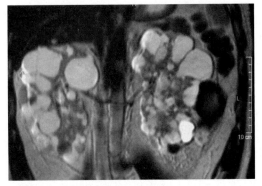

**FIGURE 2. Polycystic Kidney Disease.** Coronal T2-weighted MR image shows enlarged bilateral kidneys with numerous high signal intensity cysts.

# RENAL ARTERY STENOSIS

**Description:** The most common cause of correctable hypertension is stenosis of the renal artery. Hypertension of the renal artery can occur as a result of either atherosclerosis or fibromuscular dysplasia.

**Etiology:** Results from the accumulation of atherosclerotic plaques or fibromuscular dysplasia in the renal artery.

**Epidemiology:** Hypertension from renal artery stenosis occurs in less than 5 percent of all patients with hypertension. Atherosclerosis occurs mainly in older people. Fibromuscular dysplasia is more commonly seen in young females than young males.

**Signs and Symptoms:** Patients present with hypertension.

**Imaging Characteristics:** Noninvasive studies include captopril renal nuclear medicine scan and magnetic resonance angiography (MRA) with gadolinium. Conventional angiography is the gold standard, but it is invasive.

## CT and MRI
- Atherosclerotic narrowing involves the proximal renal artery close to its origin.
- Fibromuscular dysplasia causes a beading (string of pearls) appearance and involves the distal two-thirds of the renal artery as well as other peripheral branches.

**Treatment:** Methods of treatment include angioplasty, stenting, and surgical revascularization.

**Prognosis:** Good with early diagnosis and treatment.

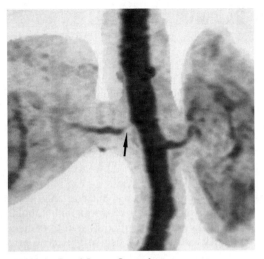

**FIGURE 1. Renal Artery Stenosis.** MRA of the abdominal aorta shows severe narrowing (*arrow*) of the proximal right renal artery close to its origin from the aorta. Left renal artery is normal.

# RENAL CALCULUS

**Description:** Renal calculi (kidney stones) may form anywhere throughout the urinary tract. They usually develop in the renal pelvis or the calyces of the kidneys. The majority of renal stones are composed of calcium salts. Kidney stones vary in size and may be solitary or multiple. They may remain in the renal pelvis or enter the ureter.

**Etiology:** Although the exact cause is unknown, predisposing factors include dehydration (increased concentration of calculus-forming substances), infection (changes in pH), obstruction (urinary stasis, such as may be seen in spinal cord injuries), and metabolic disorders (e.g., hyperparathyroidism), renal tubular acidosis, elevated uric acid (usually without gout), defective metabolism of oxalate, genetic defect in metabolism of cystine, and excessive intake of vitamin D or dietary calcium.

**Epidemiology:** Renal calculi result in roughly 1 per 1000 hospitalizations annually. They typically occur between 30 and 50 years of age. Most occur in the third decade of life. Calcium stones affect males more than females by a ratio of 3:1.

**Signs and Symptoms:** Patients may present with back pain (renal colic), pain radiating into groin area, hematuria, dysuria polyuria, chills, and fever associated with infection caused by obstruction, nausea, vomiting, diarrhea, abdominal distention, and costovertebral angle tenderness.

**Imaging Characteristics:** Noncontrast CT of the abdomen and pelvis is the imaging modality of choice and is gradually replacing the intravenous pyelogram (IVP).

## CT
- Noncontrast CT demonstrates calcified stone in the kidney or ureter.
- May show hydronephrosis and hydroureter.
- May show perinephric soft-tissue stranding.

**Treatment:** Treatment includes pain management, fluid management, straining urine for urine analysis and stone collection, and extracorporeal shock wave lithotripsy. Surgery is rarely indicated.

**Prognosis:** A good prognosis is expected with complete return to the patient's previous state of health.

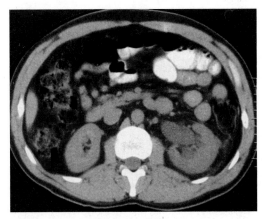

**FIGURE 1. Kidney Hydronephrosis.** CT of the abdomen without IV contrast demonstrates mild left hydronephrosis. There is left perinephric soft-tissue stranding.

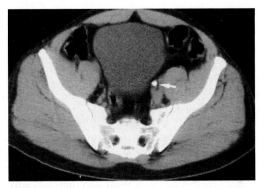

**FIGURE 2. Kidney Calculus.** CT of the pelvis on the same patient as in Figure 1, demonstrating a calcified stone (*arrow*) of the left distal ureter.

# RENAL CELL CARCINOMA

**Description:**   Renal cell carcinoma (RCC) is the most common malignancy affecting the kidney.

**Etiology:**  Although the cause of renal cell carcinoma is unknown, it is known to arise from the proximal convoluted tubule.

**Epidemiology:**   Approximately 30,000 new cases are diagnosed annually with about 12,000 deaths. Males are affected more than females at a ratio of 2:1. The average age of occurrence appears between the fifth and sixth decade of life.

**Signs and Symptoms:**  Patients may present with a solid renal mass (6 to 7 cm), hematuria, abdominal mass, anemia, flank pain, hypertension, and weight loss.

## Imaging Characteristics:
### CT
• Precontrast studies show hypodense or isodense renal mass.
• Post-IV contrast study shows enhancing mass.

### MRI
• T1-weighted images appear isointense.
• T2-weighted images appear hyperintense to parenchyma.
• Postcontrast T1-weighted images appear hyperintense with heterogeneous enhancement.

**Treatment:**  Surgical removal of the kidney (nephrectomy) when the cancer is confined to only one kidney. Radiation and chemotherapy are of little value in treating RCC.

**Prognosis:**  Depends on the staging at the time of diagnosis.

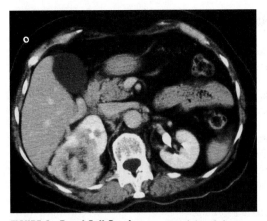

**FIGURE 1.  Renal Cell Carcinoma.**  CT of the abdomen with IV contrast demonstrates a large solid round mass of the posterior aspect of the right kidney. Note the low-density areas within the mass, which are consistent with necrosis. There is also some contrast enhancement.

# RENAL INFARCT

**Description:**  A renal infarct is a localized area of necrosis in the kidney.

**Etiology:**  An acute infarct of the kidney may follow a thromboembolic (most common), renal artery occlusion (caused by atherosclerosis), blunt abdominal trauma, or a sudden, complete renal venous occlusion.

**Epidemiology:**  The most common cause of renal emboli occurs in patients with atrial arrhythmias or have a history of a myocardial infarction. In addition, patients who have experienced blunt abdominal trauma (the kidney is the most commonly affected abdominal organ) may develop renal emboli.

**Signs and Symptoms:**  This condition may go unnoticed; some patients, however, may experience pain with tenderness in the region of the costovertebral angle of the affected side.

**Imaging Characteristics:**  Contrast-enhanced CT is the preferred modality. Convention renal arteriogram is the gold standard for the evaluation of an occlusion of renal artery or its branches.

## CT
- Contrast enhanced images show a wedge-shaped hypodense area as the affected region.

## MRI
- T1- and T2-weighted images may demonstrate a lower than normal signal in the affected area.
- T1-weighted postcontrast images demonstrate a wedge-shaped low signal area of the renal parenchyma.
- Magnetic resonance angiography may show occlusion of the main renal artery or its branches.

**Treatment:**  Thrombectomy or embolectomy may be useful in the early stage.

**Prognosis:**  Depends on early detection and treatment.

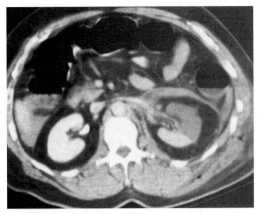

**FIGURE 1. Renal Infarct Secondary to Emboli.**
Contrast-enhanced CT of the abdomen shows hypodense area (no perfusion) of the anterior aspect of the left kidney.

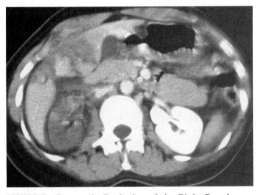

**FIGURE 2. Traumatic Occlusion of the Right Renal Artery.** Contrast-enhanced CT of the abdomen shows absent parenchymal enhancement of the right kidney, consistent with a total infarction.

# INFECTION

## APPENDICITIS

**Description:**   Appendicitis is the inflammation of the vermiform appendix because of an obstruction. Appendicitis is the most common acute surgical condition of the abdomen.

**Etiology:**   Obstruction of the vermiform appendix.

**Epidemiology:**   Appendicitis can occur at any age and affects males and females equally.

**Signs and Symptoms:**   Patient may present with abdominal pain or tenderness in the right lower quadrant (McBurney point), anorexia, nausea and vomiting, and constipation.

**Imaging Characteristics:**   CT exam may be performed either with or without IV contrast. No oral contrast is needed.

**CT**
- Dilated, fluid-filled appendix.
- May present with a calcified appendicolith.
- Ring-like enhancement with contrast.
- Associated with periappendiceal inflammation or abscess.

**Treatment:**   Immediate surgical intervention (appendectomy) is required.

**Prognosis:**   Usually uncomplicated course of recovery in nonruptured appendicitis. If the appendix ruptures, there is a variable degree of morbidity and mortality based on the age of the patient.

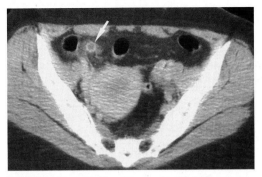

**FIGURE 1. Appendicitis.** IV contrast CT demonstrates round tubular structure with ring-like peripheral enhancement (*arrow*) in the right lower quadrant with periappendiceal soft-tissue stranding representing inflammation.

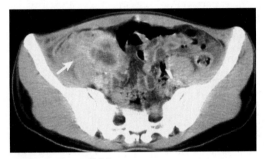

**FIGURE 2. Appendicitis.** CT with IV contrast shows inflammatory mass or abscess in the right lower quadrant secondary to ruptured appendix. (*arrow*)

# DIVERTICULITIS

**Description:**   Diverticulitis is a complication of diverticulosis. Diverticulitis is an abscess or inflammation initiated by the rupture of the diverticula into the pericolic fat.

**Etiology:**   Diverticulitis is a secondary complication to ruptured diverticula.

**Epidemiology:**   Diverticulosis rarely affects those younger than 40 years of age. Approximately 40 to 50 percent of the general population is affected by the time persons reach their sixth to eighth decades of life.

**Signs and Symptoms:**  Pain is most commonly seen in the left lower quadrant. The patient usually experiences either diarrhea or constipation. When considering diverticulitis, in addition to the above, patients will experience fever with chills, anorexia, nausea and vomiting, and tenderness in the left lower quadrant.

## Imaging Characteristics:

### CT
- Early signs of diverticulitis include wispy, streaky densities in the pericolic fat, and a slight thickening of the colon wall.
- Severe cases of diverticulitis may demonstrate pericolic abscesses.

**Treatment:** Usually treated with IV antibiotics. Abscess may require CT-guided catheter drainage or surgical intervention.

**Prognosis:**  With early detection and treatment the patient should experience a good recovery.

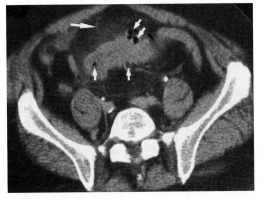

**FIGURE 1. Diverticulitis.** CT of the pelvis with IV contrast demonstrates multiple (*short arrows*) diverticula in the sigmoid colon. There is soft-tissue stranding (*long arrow*) of the pericolic fat. There is no evidence of fluid collection or abscess.

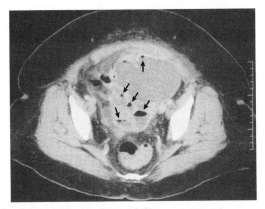

**FIGURE 2. Diverticulitis with Abscess.** CT of the pelvis with IV contrast demonstrates a large round fluid collection in the left pelvis. There are a few air bubbles (*arrows*) within the fluid collect. These findings are consistent with an abscess.

# PERINEPHRIC ABSCESS

**Description:** A perinephric abscess is a collection of pus within the fatty tissue around the kidney.

**Etiology:** Results from a bacterial infection such as *Escherichia coli* and *Proteus* and *Staphylococcus* in a few cases.

**Epidemiology:** Perinephric abscesses usually arise from a preexisting renal inflammatory disease. However, they may occur a complication of surgery, trauma, or spread from other organs.

**Signs and Symptoms:** Patients will present with flank or back pain, fever, nausea and vomiting, malaise, and painful urination.

**Imaging Characteristics:** Contrast-enhanced CT is the modality of choice for the diagnosis.

## CT
- Abscess appears with lower than normal attenuation (hypodense) values when compared to normal parenchyma.
- Rim enhancement of the abscess occurs with administration of IV contrast.
- Stranding densities in the perirenal fat and thickening of the renal fascia.
- Gas pockets may be seen within the abscess.

**Treatment:** Intravenous administration of antibiotics and percutaneous catheter drainage. Surgery is rarely needed.

**Prognosis:** Generally good with early diagnosis and treatment.

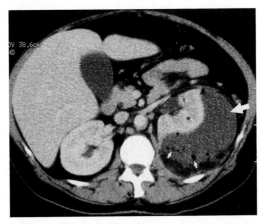

**FIGURE 1. Left Perinephric Abscess.** Contrast CT of the abdomen shows a large fluid collection (*thick arrow*) around the left kidney (*asterisk*). Note the gas bubbles within the fluid collection (*small arrows*).

# RENAL ABSCESS

**Description:** A renal abscess is a collection of pus within the parenchyma of the kidney.

**Etiology:** Results from a bacterial infection.

**Epidemiology:** Most renal abscesses are the result of an ascending infection and are usually caused by gram-negative urinary pathogens, particularly *E. coli*. To a lesser degree renal abscesses may be a consequence of a complication from surgery, trauma, spread from other organs, or lymphatic spread.

**Signs and Symptoms:** Patients will present with flank or back pain, fever, nausea and vomiting, malaise, and painful urination.

**Imaging Characteristics:** Contrast-enhanced CT is the modality of choice for the diagnosis.

## CT
- Abscess appears with lower than normal attenuation (hypodense) values when compared to normal parenchyma.
- Rim enhancement of the abscess occurs with administration of IV contrast.
- Stranding densities in the perirenal fat and thickening of the renal fascia.
- Gas pockets may be seen within the abscess.

**Treatment:** Intravenous administration of antibiotics and percutaneous catheter drainage. Surgery is rarely needed.

**Prognosis:** Generally good with early diagnosis and treatment.

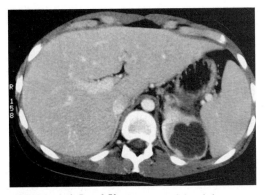

**FIGURE 1. Left Renal Abscess.** CT of the abdomen with IV contrast demonstrates a round low-density mass in the upper pole of the left kidney. Ultrasound showed this mass to be complex. Combination of these findings in a patient with flank pain, fever, and leukocytosis is consistent with a renal abscess.

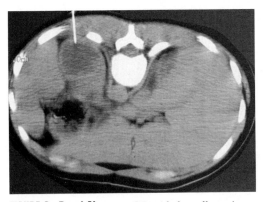

**FIGURE 2. Renal Abscess**. CT-guided needle aspiration of a cystic mass in the upper pole of the left kidney yielded pus. The aspirating needle is within the abscess. This abscess was successfully treated with catheter drainage and antibiotics. Note the patient is in the prone position.

# TRAUMA

## LIVER LACERATION

**Description:** Lacerations to the liver can occur as a result of blunt or penetrating abdominal trauma, as a complication of surgery, or an interventional procedure.

**Etiology:** A laceration to the liver usually results from an injury such as blunt or penetrating abdominal trauma. However, complication of surgery or an interventional procedure can also result in a laceration type injury.

**Epidemiology:** Trauma to the abdomen results in approximately 10 percent of all traumatic deaths. Many of these injuries occur as secondary injuries as a result of high-speed motor vehicle accidents.

**Signs and Symptoms:** Abdominal pain resulting from the blunt trauma or an open wound occurring from a penetrating injury. The patient may experience hypovolemic shock that is caused from an inadequate blood volume.

**Imaging Characteristics:** CT with IV contrast is the imaging modality of choice in the evaluation of abdominal trauma.

### CT
- A noncontrast study may not reveal the injury.
- Contrast enhancement will assist in demonstrating the laceration as a hypodense area.
- May show subcapsular hematoma.
- May show hemoperitoneum.

**Treatment:** Emergency surgical intervention may be required to repair the laceration of the liver in hemodynamically unstable patients. Stable patients with small lacerations can be treated conservatively.

**Prognosis:** Depends on the severity of the injury and associated injuries to other organs.

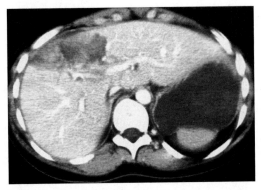

**FIGURE 1. Liver Laceration.** CT of the abdomen with IV contrast demonstrates a large hypodense area of the anterior aspect of the right lobe of the liver consistent with a laceration and hematoma.

# SPLENIC LACERATION

**Description:** The spleen is the most commonly injured abdominal organ. Injury to the spleen can occur as a result of blunt or penetrating trauma to the abdomen.

**Etiology:** Injuries such as lacerations occur as a result of blunt or penetrating trauma to the abdominal region.

**Epidemiology:** The spleen is the most commonly injured abdominal organ.

**Signs and Symptoms:** Depending on the degree of the injury and other related injuries, the patient would probably present with abdominal pain, possible open wound, and symptoms associated with hypovolemic shock (i.e., low blood pressure and rapid pulse).

**Imaging Characteristics:** CT of the abdomen with IV contrast is the best way to evaluate splenic injuries and also to evaluate to other viscera.

## CT
- Noncontrast CT may not demonstrate a hematoma or laceration.
- IV contrast CT shows an irregular linear hypodensity of a splenic laceration and perisplenic hematoma. There may also be a hemoperitoneum (blood in the peritoneal cavity).

**Treatment:** Depending on the extent of the injury, surgical intervention may be required.

**Prognosis:** Excluding other related injuries that may be associated with the splenic laceration, patient recovery is encouraging.

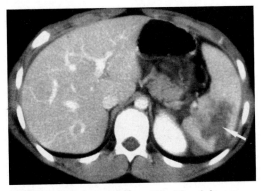

**FIGURE 1. Splenic Laceration.** CT of the abdomen with IV contrast shows low-density areas (*arrow*) within the posterior aspect of the spleen consistent with a deep laceration and hematomas.

# MISCELLANEOUS

## AORTIC ANEURYSM

**Description:** An abdominal aortic aneurysm (AAA) is a permanent, abnormal, localized dilatation of the aorta.

**Etiology:** Approximately 95 percent of abdominal aortic aneurysms result from a weakening of the arterial wall as a result of atherosclerosis.

**Epidemiology:** Men are affected more than females by a ratio of 3:1. Usually arises between 60 and 80 years of age. Incidence rate is roughly 1 in 10,000 patients admitted to hospitals. With approximately 15,000 deaths yearly, this is the tenth leading cause of death in males older than age 55 years.

**Signs and Symptoms:** Abdominal aneurysms are generally asymptomatic. The most common evidence includes a pulsating mass in the periumbilical area, accompanied by systolic bruit over the aorta with back and abdominal pain.

**Imaging Characteristics:** Ultrasound is good for screening. CT with IV contrast is better for evaluation of the aortic aneurysm.

### CT
- Demonstrates the location, size and shape of the aneurysm.
- May show intramural thrombus within the aneurysm.

### MRI
- Same findings as CT.
- Magnetic resonance angiography (MRA) with IV contrast is used to evaluate the extent of the aneurysm and its relationship to the renal arteries.

**Treatment:** An aortic aneurysm greater than 5 cm or progressively increasing in size is an indication for surgery.

**Prognosis:** If the aneurysm is diagnosed and treated prior to rupture, the prognosis is favorable. A ruptured aneurysm has a high mortality rate.

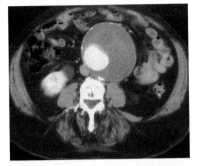

**FIGURE 1. Abdominal Aortic Aneurysm.** CT of the abdomen with IV contrast in a patient demonstrating a very large fusiform abdominal aortic aneurysm with a large intramural thrombus and small contrast opacified patent lumen.

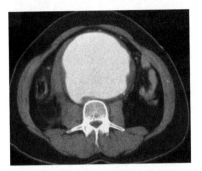

**FIGURE 2. Abdominal Aortic Aneurysm.** CT of the abdomen with IV contrast demonstrates a huge abdominal aortic aneurysm with contrast opacified lumen.

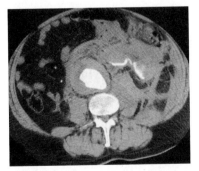

**FIGURE 3. Ruptured Abdominal Aortic Aneurysm.** CT of the abdomen with IV contrast demonstrates a ruptured abdominal aortic aneurysm with a large left retroperitoneal hematoma. Note leakage of contrast into the retroperitoneal hematoma, indicating an active bleed.

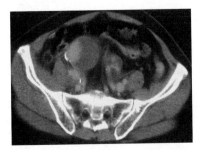

**FIGURE 4. Right Iliac Artery Aneurysm.** CT of the pelvis without IV contrast demonstrates a large right iliac artery aneurysm with calcification in the wall and intramural thrombus measuring close to 5 cm.

# LYMPHOMA

**Description:** Lymphomas are malignant tumors involving the lymphatic system. Lymphomas are usually grouped into two groups: (1) Hodgkin's disease and (2) non-Hodgkin's lymphoma (NHL). As a result of its characteristic pathology (i.e., Reed-Sternberg cell), Hodgkin's disease is considered separately. All other malignant lymphomas are grouped under the term non-Hodgkin's lymphoma.

**Etiology:** Although the cause of malignant lymphomas is unknown, viral involvement, such as with the Epstein-Barr virus, is suspected.

**Epidemiology:** Approximately 45,000 new cases are diagnosed annually with slightly more than 50 percent being males. The incidence rises with age, with a median age of 50 years.

**Signs and Symptoms:** Similar to Hodgkin's disease. Usually involves swelling or enlargement of lymphoid tissue and glands and is painless. Symptoms develop specific to the area involved and systemic complaints of fatigue, malaise, weight loss, fever, and night sweats may be experienced.

**Imaging Characteristics:** CT is the preferred modality for the diagnosis and staging of lymphoma.

## CT
- Used in the staging of lymphomas.
- Can also be used for CT-guided needle biopsies of lymphomas.
- Demonstrates enlarged retroperitoneal, paraaortic and paracaval lymph nodes.
- Demonstrates enlarged mesenteric lymph nodes.
- Demonstrates enlarged liver and spleen.

**Treatment:** Radiation therapy and chemotherapy are used to treat non-Hodgkin's lymphomas. Surgery is primarily used in establishing the diagnosis and assisting with anatomic staging.

**Prognosis:** Depends on the cell type and extent of the disease. Hodgkin's disease usually has a better prognosis.

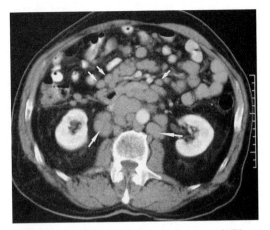

**FIGURE 1. Lymphoma.** CT of the abdomen with IV contrast demonstrates multiple enlarged retroperitoneal paraaortic and paracaval lymph nodes (*long arrows*), as well as enlarged mesenteric lymph nodes (*short arrows*).

# SOFT-TISSUE SARCOMA

**Description:** Soft-tissue sarcomas of the body consist of a group of malignant tumors that originate in the connective tissues. Sarcomas are named according to the specific type of tissue they affect.

**Etiology:** It is not known how soft-tissue sarcomas develop. There is some evidence that soft-tissue sarcomas can be influenced by genetics; occupational exposure to certain chemicals used in the agricultural, forestry, and railroad industries; exposure of Vietnam veterans to the herbicide "Agent Orange" which contains dioxin; and exposure to radiation. There is a latency period associated with the occurrence of soft-tissue sarcomas that seems to exist over the course of several years.

**Epidemiology:** Soft-tissue sarcomas account for approximately 1 percent of all malignant tumors found in adults. Roughly 6,000 new cases are diagnosed annually with approximately 3,300 deaths. Males and females seem to be equally affected. Whites are more affected (90 percent) than blacks (6 percent), and other races contribute to the remaining 4 percent.

**Signs and Symptoms:** The signs and symptoms may vary depending on the soft-tissue structure affected. Some patients may present with a palpable mass. Some patients experience pain, while other patients are asymptomatic.

## Imaging Characteristics:

### CT
- May appear as a solid, mixed, or pseudocystic mass.
- Enhancement with IV contrast may be variable.

### MRI
- Signal intensity may be homogeneous or heterogeneous and appear as a mass.
- The type of tissue involved will affect the signal intensity.

**Treatment:** Surgical intervention with radiation and chemotherapy are used in the treatment of soft-tissue sarcomas.

**Prognosis:** Depends on the tumor size and anatomic location, histologic grade, and extent of spread to adjacent tissues and distant metastases. The 5-year survival rate ranges from 30 percent to 90 percent. As with all malignant tumors, the earlier the cancer is detected and treatment begun, the better the prognosis.

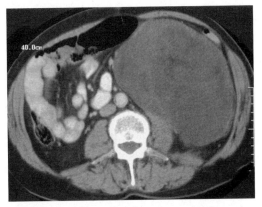

**FIGURE 1. Soft-Tissue Sarcoma.** Contrast-enhanced CT of the abdomen shows large soft-tissue mass occupying most of the left abdomen displacing bowel loops to the right. There is no significant contrast enhancement.

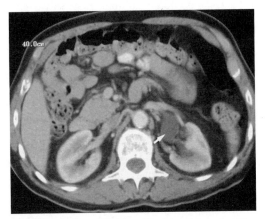

**FIGURE 2. Hydronephrosis.** CT of the abdomen with contrast shows hydronephrosis of the left kidney (*arrow*) secondary to obstruction of the left distal ureter by the left-sided abdominal mass.

# SMALL-BOWEL OBSTRUCTION

**Description:** Obstruction of the small bowel is one of the most common causes of abdominal pain.

**Etiology:** Adhesions that have formed as a result of previous abdominal surgery are the most common cause of small-bowel obstruction (SBO). Other extrinsic causes of SBO include malignant tumor, hernia, volvulus, abscess or hematoma. Intrinsic factors, which occur less often, include neoplasm, inflammatory bowel disease, ischemic bowel disease, and intussusception.

**Epidemiology:** Males and females are equally affected. Small-bowel obstruction can occur at any age.

**Signs and Symptoms:** Obstruction of the bowel typically causes pain, vomiting, distention, and constipation.

**Imaging Characteristics:** Plain films (supine and upright) are helpful in most cases and should be done first. However, uncertain findings (i.e., false-positive and false-negative studies) occur in as many as 50 percent of the patients. CT is very accurate in diagnosing SBO (70 to 100 percent). CT can identify the cause of the obstruction in (50 to 85 percent) of the patients imaged.

## CT

- Shows dilated loops of the small bowel (2.5 cm or greater in diameter).
- Point of transition distal to where the small bowel and colon are collapsed.
- Can diagnose closed loop obstruction (i.e., strangulation), which is usually caused by ischemia and infarction.
- Preferable to use IV contrast. If oral contrast is needed, a water-soluble oral contrast is preferred.

**Treatment:** Surgical intervention to correct the causative agent.

**Prognosis:** Depends on the causative agent and other patient related factors such as the patient's overall health.

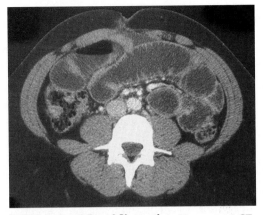

**FIGURE 1. Small-Bowel Obstruction.** Noncontrast CT of the abdomen shows moderately dilated fluid-filled small bowel consistent with a mechanical obstruction.

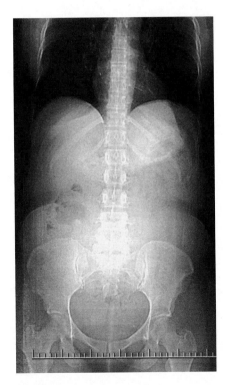

**FIGURE 2. Small-Bowel Obstruction.** CT scout image of the same patient is unremarkable. There is no evidence of dilated small bowel. Note that if the dilated small bowel contains only fluid and no air, plain films may appear normal in small-bowel obstruction. CT is useful in imaging these patients.

# SPLENOMEGALY

**Description:**  Splenomegaly is an abnormal enlargement of the spleen.

**Etiology:**  Splenomegaly may be associated with numerous conditions, including a neoplasm, abscess, cyst, infection, portal hypertension (cirrhosis), and hematologic disorders (hemolytic anemia and leukemia).

**Epidemiology:**  Patients with any of the above conditions may develop an enlarged spleen.

**Signs and Symptoms:** Depends on the causative agent. A palpable mass may be detected in some cases, while splenomegaly may be an incidental finding.

## Imaging Characteristics:

### CT and MRI
- Shows enlarged spleen.
- Focal lesions may be present.
- Displacement of adjacent organs may be seen.

**Treatment:**  Depends on the causative agent. Surgery may be required.

**Prognosis:**  Depends on the etiology.

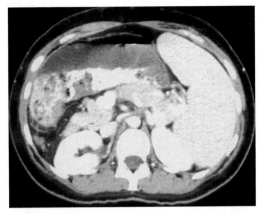

**FIGURE 1. Splenomegaly.** CT of the abdomen with contrast demonstrates an enlarged spleen extending inferiorly into the lower abdomen displacing the left kidney medially.

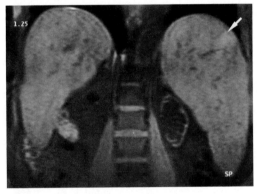

**FIGURE 2. Splenomegaly.** Coronal gradient echo MRI of the abdomen demonstrates an enlarged spleen (*arrow*).

# PART VI

# Pelvis

# ADENOMYOSIS

**Description:** Adenomyosis is the presence of endometrium inside the myometrium.

**Etiology:** Adenomyosis is most likely a result of direct invasion of the endometrium into the myometrium.

**Epidemiology:** The exact incidence rate is unknown. It is most commonly detected during the fifth decade of life. Adenomyosis is present in 8 to 20 percent of hysterectomy specimens.

**Signs and Symptoms:** Patient presents with pelvic pain, menorrhagia, an enlarged uterus or a combination of the above. Some patients may be asymptomatic.

**Imaging Characteristics:** MRI is the imaging modality of choice for the diagnosis of adenomyosis. Historically, prior to MRI, adenomyosis was diagnosed by hysterectomy.

## MRI
- Thickening either even or uneven (> 5 mm) of the junctional zone (JZ).
- Low-signal intensity on T1- and T2-weighted images.
- T1-weighted images may show small high signal intensities representing small foci of hemorrhage.
- T2-weighted images show an ill-defined, poorly marginated area of low-signal intensity within the myometrium but contiguous with the JZ.

**Treatment:** A hysterectomy is the treatment of choice.

**Prognosis:** Good; this is a benign lesion.

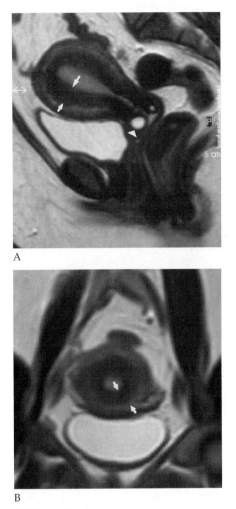

A

B

**FIGURE 1 Adenomyosis.** T2-weighted sagittal (A) and axial (B) images demonstrate (1 cm) thickening of the junctional (dark area) zone (*arrows*) surrounding the endometrial cavity (bright area) consistent with adenomyosis. Incidental finding of a nabothian cyst of the cervix (*arrowhead*).

# UTERINE LEIOMYOMA: (FIBROID UTERUS)

**Description:**   Uterine leiomyomas, also known as myomas, fibromyomas, and fibroids are the most common benign uterine tumor.

**Etiology:**   The cause is unknown. A leiomyoma is an estrogen-dependent tumor that may increase in size during pregnancy, and usually decreases in size following menopause.

**Epidemiology:**  Leiomyomas occur in 20 to 30 percent of premenopausal women. Black women are affected three times more then white women.

**Signs and Symptoms:**  Depending on the location and size of the tumor, the patient may experience pressure on the surrounding organs and abnormal menstruation.

**Imaging Characteristics:**  Ultrasound is the best imaging modality.

## CT
- Usually appear with a homogenous soft-tissue density similar to a normal uterus.
- Calcification may occur in approximately 10 percent of cases, especially postmenopausal patients.
- Contrast-enhanced images demonstrates enhancement similar to a normal uterus.

## MRI
- T1- and T2-weighted images show masses of mixed signal intensity.
- T1-weighted images demonstrate acute hemorrhage as increased signal intensity.
- Multiplanar imaging is very useful for the evaluation of the size and location of the fibroids in young the patient for myomectomy planning.

**Treatment:**  Myomectomy in the young reproductive age group. Hysterectomy for older and severe cases. Uterine artery embolization also may be used to treat the fibroids.

**Prognosis:**  Good; these tumors are benign.

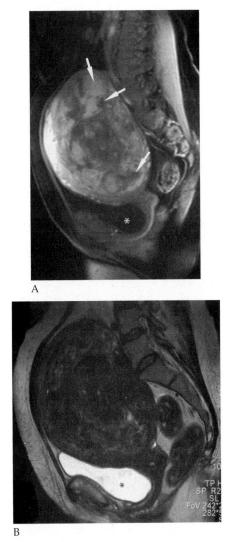

A

B

**FIGURE 1. Fibroid Uterus.** Proton density
(A) and T2-weighted (B) sagittal MR images
demonstrate diffusely enlarged uterus
compressing the bladder (*asterisk*). There are
multiple masses of various signal intensities
(*arrows*) of the uterus, seen better on proton
density images.

# OVARIAN CYST

**Description:** An adnexal mass of the uterus can comprise any of the appendages of the uterus including the ovaries, fallopian tubes and the ligaments that hold the uterus in place. The majority of cysts and tumors affecting the ovaries are benign, well-circumscribed, round, near-water density with a cyst wall that is difficult to see.

**Etiology:** Generally related to hormonal dysfunction however may be stimulated by other disease processes.

**Epidemiology:** Occurs more commonly in menarcheal women.

**Signs and Symptoms:** Adnexal cysts are usually asymptomatic.

**Imaging Characteristics:** Ultrasound is the best modality for imaging of the uterus and ovaries.

## CT
- Contrast-enhanced CT demonstrates a cystic mass in the adnexal region.
- Well-defined margins with fluid density.

## MRI
- T1-weighted image shows the cyst with low signal intensity.
- T2-weighted image shows the cyst with high signal intensity.

**Treatment:** Surgery may be required for larger (>5 cm) cysts.

**Prognosis:** Good; this is a benign cyst.

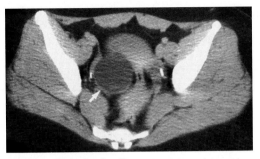

**FIGURE 1. Right Ovarian Cyst.** CT of the pelvis with contrast shows an approximate 5-cm round, well-defined, low-density mass (*arrow*) in the right adnexal consistent with an ovarian cyst.

# PART VII

---

# Musculoskeletal

---

# SHOULDER

## HILL-SACHS DEFECT

**Description:** A Hill-Sachs defect is an impaction (compression) fracture of the posterosuperior and lateral aspects of the humeral head. This is usually associated with an anterior dislocation of the shoulder.

**Etiology:** A Hill-Sachs defect occurs when the shoulder is traumatically abducted and externally rotated compressing the posterior aspect of the humeral head against the glenoid rim. This force may produce an impaction (compression) fracture of the humeral head characteristic of the injury.

**Epidemiology:** The associated impaction fracture seen in a Hill-Sachs defect occurs in approximately 60 percent of the population diagnosed with an anterior dislocation of the shoulder.

**Signs and Symptoms:** Pain, stiffness, shoulder instability, avascular necrosis, and posttraumatic myositis ossificans may accompany this injury.

### Imaging Characteristics:

### CT
- Reveals the compression fracture associated with injury to the posteriolateral aspect of the humeral head resulting from an anterior dislocation of the shoulder. Hill-Sachs defect is best seen at the level of the coracoid.

### MRI
- Appear as wedge-like defects on the posteriolateral aspect of the humeral head.
- T1-weighted images show the low-signal injury.
- T2-weighted images depict the injury as hyperintense.
- STIR images are more sensitive for the diagnosis of subtle fracture or of a bone bruise that appears with a high signal.
- MR arthrography is excellent for the evaluation of tears of the glenoid labrum in patients with recurrent shoulder dislocation.

**Treatment:** Surgical intervention may be required for recurrent shoulder dislocation.

**Prognosis:** Results may vary depending on extenuating circumstances, however, the patient is encouraged to gradually resume normal use.

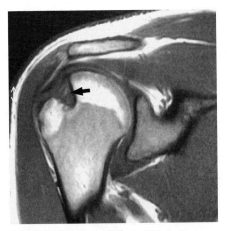

**FIGURE 1. Hill-Sachs Defect.** Hill-Sachs defect seen in a patient with a history of an anterior dislocation of the shoulder. T1-weighted oblique coronal image of the shoulder demonstrates a wedge shaped defect in the superior lateral aspect of the head of the humerus (*arrow*) consistent with a Hill-Sachs defect.

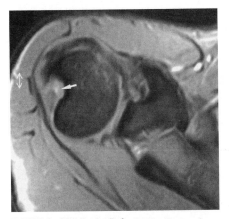

**FIGURE 2. Hill-Sachs Defect.** Gradient echo axial image of the shoulder demonstrates a wedge shaped defect (*arrow*) along the posterior lateral aspect of the head of the humerus consistent with a Hill-Sachs defect.

# ROTATOR CUFF TEAR

**Description:** The rotator cuff of the shoulder is comprised of a thick, tough, tendinous capsule surrounding the four tendons representing the insertions of the supraspinatus, infraspinatus, the teres minor muscles (insert into the greater tuberosity and assist with external rotation) and the subscapularis (inserts into the lesser tuberosity and assist with internal rotation). Tearing of the rotator cuff can be categorized as partial or complete tears.

**Etiology:** Usually results from chronic degenerative impingement. Other causes may include acute and chronic trauma. Sports and occupational overuse may also be associated with rotator cuff tears.

**Epidemiology:** Injury involving the rotator cuff is one of the most common causes of shoulder pain and disability.

**Signs and Symptoms:** Progressive pain and weakness accompanying a loss of motion. Shoulder pain increases when performing activities at or above the level of the shoulder. Night pain is often experienced.

**Imaging Characteristics:** MRI has completely replaced shoulder arthrography.

## MRI
- T2-weighted fat saturated images shows the tear as high signal.
- There may be discontinuity and retraction of the rotator cuff tendons.
- Fluid in the subacromial/subdeltoid bursa.
- Superior migration of the head of the humerus.
- Degenerative hypertrophy of the acromioclavicular (AC) joint.
- MR arthrography is also useful for the evaluation of labral tears.

**Treatment:** Depends on the severity of the injury. Early diagnosis, pain management, and surgical intervention may encourage better patient outcome.

**Prognosis:** Patient outcome varies depending on degree of the injury, method of treatment, patient discomfort level with pain, and shoulder mobility.

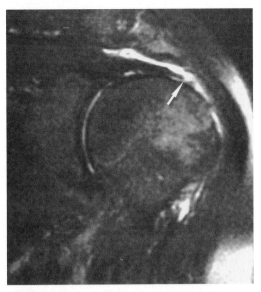

**FIGURE 1. Rotator Cuff Tear.** T2-weighted oblique coronal MRI with fat suppression shows a full-thickness tear (*arrow*) of the distal rotator cuff tendon (supraspinatus muscle) with some medial retraction. A small amount of fluid is in the subacromial/subdeltoid bursa.

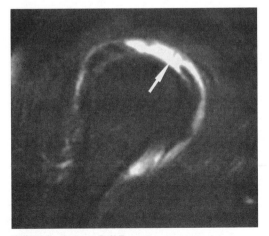

**FIGURE 2. Rotator Cuff Tear.** Fat-suppressed T2-weighted oblique sagittal image demonstrates a full thickness tear (*arrow*) of the rotator cuff with fluid in the subacromial/ subdeltoid bursa.

# ELBOW

## TRICEPS TENDON TEAR

**Description:** The triceps tendon is the least common of all tendons in the body to rupture and is an uncommon cause of posterior elbow pain. Tearing of the triceps tendon can be classified as partial or complete. A complete tearing of the triceps tendon is uncommon and partial tears are even less common. The tendon will typically rupture at its attachment near the olecranon.

**Etiology:** A rupture of the triceps tendon usually occurs as a result of direct blow to the tendon, a fall on an outstretched arm or a decelerating counterforce during active extension. In some cases, the tendon may undergo degeneration or erosion in association with olecranon bursitis.

**Epidemiology:** The triceps tendon is the least common of all tendons in the body to rupture.

**Signs and Symptoms:** Patient presents with posterior elbow pain.

**Imaging Characteristics:** MRI is the imaging modality of choice.

### MRI
- Axial and sagittal imaging are necessary to evaluate partial versus complete tear and size of the gap associated with the tear. This information is useful in preoperative planning.
- Abnormal increased signal may be seen in the tendon in a partial tear or tendinopathy.
- Discontinuous fibers are noted with complete tear.
- Most tears occur at the insertion on to the olecranon.

**Treatment:** Surgical repair is required as soon as possible.

**Prognosis:** In general, the results are good.

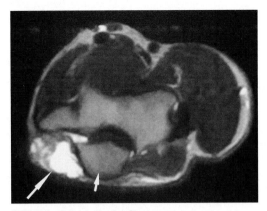

**FIGURE 1. Triceps Tendon Tear.** T2-weighted axial MRI shows increased signal intensity within the distal triceps tendon (*long arrow*) near its insertion to the olecranon process of the ulnar (*short arrow*).

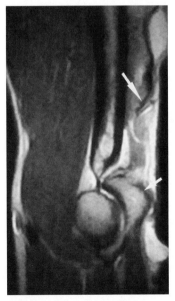

**FIGURE 2. Triceps Tendon Tear.** Sagittal T2-weighted MRI shows a completely torn and retracted triceps tendon (*long arrow*) from the olecranon (*short arrow*).

# HAND AND WRIST

## GANGLION CYST

**Description:** A ganglion is a small (1.0 to 2.0-cm) benign cyst that may be seen around any joint capsule or tendon sheath. Ganglions are commonly located around the joints of the wrist.

**Etiology:** Although there is no known cause for the development of ganglions, it is suspected that they are caused by a coalescence of small cysts formed as a result of degeneration of periarticular connective tissue.

**Epidemiology:** Ganglions typically present between the second and fourth decades of life. There is a slight female predominance.

**Signs and Symptoms:** These firm, movable lesions are often asymptomatic. Ganglions that occur in the carpal tunnel or Guyon canal may cause compression of the median and ulnar nerves, respectively.

**Imaging Characteristics:**

### CT
- Round, low-density mass with fluid attenuation value.

### MRI
- A ganglion is usually a round, lobulated, homogeneous mass with low signal on T1-weighted images.
- This cystic lesion will appear hyperintense on T2-weighted images.
- Postcontrast T1-weighted images will not enhance.

**Treatment:** Surgical excision of the ganglion cyst.

**Prognosis:** Good; this is a benign cyst.

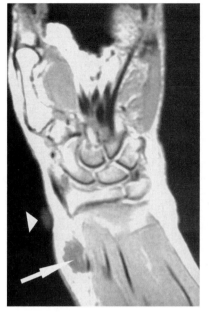

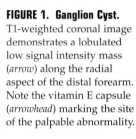

**FIGURE 1. Ganglion Cyst.**
T1-weighted coronal image demonstrates a lobulated low signal intensity mass (*arrow*) along the radial aspect of the distal forearm. Note the vitamin E capsule (*arrowhead*) marking the site of the palpable abnormality.

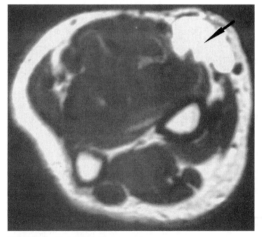

**FIGURE 2. Ganglion Cyst.** T2-weighted image demonstrates a lobulated high signal intensity mass (*arrow*) with well-defined margins consistent with a ganglion cyst along the volar radial aspect of the distal forearm close to the wrist.

# HIP

## AVASCULAR NECROSIS (OSTEONECROSIS)

**Description:** Avascular necrosis (AVN) occurs as an interruption in the blood flow within the bone (e.g., femoral head), resulting in the death of the hematopoietic cells, osteocytes, and marrow fat cells making up the bony structure.

**Etiology:** Avascular necrosis may result from trauma (fractures, dislocation), corticosteroids, Caisson disease, (in which individuals who are removed too quickly from a high pressure environment, such as in deep water diving, are prone to develop nitrogen bubbles which may cause a bony infarct), Legg-Calvé-Perthes disease, sickle cell disease, or radiation exposure, or it may be idiopathic.

**Epidemiology:** The hip is the most common site affected. Males are more affected than females by as much as a 4:1 ratio. Most patients diagnosed with (AVN) are between 30 and 70 years of age. Bilateral involvement may occur in as many 50 percent of the cases.

**Signs and Symptoms:** Increased joint pain as bone and joint begin to collapse, limited range of motion due to pain, decreased usage of the limb involved.

**Imaging Characteristics:** MRI is the most sensitive modality for the diagnosis of avascular necrosis.

### MRI
- Diffuse edema.
- Serpiginous line (low signal intensity) with a fatty center.
- Focal subchondral low signal lesion on T1-weighted images and variable signal on T2-weighted images.

**Treatment:** Treatments may include medications for pain, assistive devices to reduce weight on the bone or joint, core decompression, osteotomy, bone graft, arthroplasty (total joint replacement), electrical stimulation, or any combination of therapies to encourage the growth of new bone.

**Prognosis:**  Mixed and variable, dependent upon the underlying cause of the disease, overall health and medical history, extent of the disease, location and amount of bone affected, and tolerance to specific medications, procedures, or therapies.

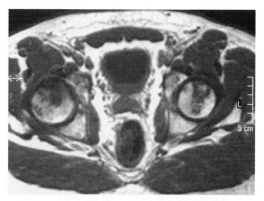

**FIGURE 1.  Avascular Necrosis of the Femoral Heads.**
T1-weighted axial MRI shows focal decreased marrow signal intensity of the femoral heads bilaterally. The right femoral head is worse than the left.

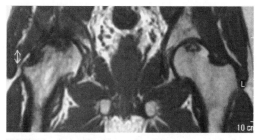

**FIGURE 2.  Avascular Necrosis of the Femoral Heads.**
T1-weighted coronal MRI shows focal decreased marrow signal intensity of the femoral heads bilaterally, worse on the right side.

# HIP DISLOCATION

**Description:** Dislocation of the hip may be associated with a fracture of the acetabulum. The acetabulum or articular socket of the hip is composed of and supported by two columns of bone. The bone of the iliac crest, iliac spines, anterior half of the acetabulum, and the pubis comprise to form the anterior column. The ischium, ischial spine, posterior half of the acetabulum, and the sciatic notch comprise to form the posterior column. The superior portion (i.e., dome or roof) of the acetabulum is the weight-bearing portion of the articular surface that supports the femoral head.

**Etiology:** Hip dislocations and fractures to the acetabulum or pelvis are commonly caused by trauma.

**Epidemiology:** Hip dislocations are frequently associated with a femoral fracture. A posterior hip dislocation, the most common type occurs in approximately 90 percent of the cases and is frequently associated with a fracture to the posterior margin of the acetabulum.

**Signs and Symptoms:** Patient presents with pain and loss of function to the extremity affected.

### Imaging Characteristics:

#### CT
- Identify intraarticular bony fragments.
- Thin-section multiplanar reconstructed sagittal and coronal images are useful.

#### MRI
- T1-weighted images appear with low signal intensity to the affected area.
- T2-weighted images appear with high signal intensity to the affected area.
- STIR images appear with high signal intensity to the affected area.
- Useful for the evaluation of avascular necrosis in the head of the femur.

**Treatment:** Depends on the extent of the injury and other related injuries. Patients will require either an open or closed reduction.

**Prognosis:** Depends on the extent of the injury and other related injuries.

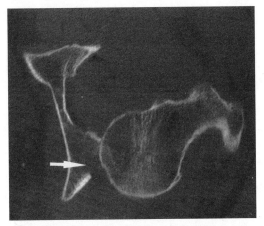

**FIGURE 1. Posterior Dislocation of the Left Hip.**
Axial CT of the hip shows a posteriorly dislocated
left femoral head. There is a fracture of the posterior
acetabulum margin (*arrow*).

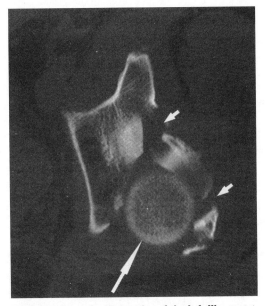

**FIGURE 2. Posterior Dislocation of the Left Hip.** Axial
CT of the left hip shows a posteriorly dislocated left
femoral head (*long arrow*) and fractures of the left
acetabulum (*short arrows*).

# KNEE

## ANTERIOR CRUCIATE LIGAMENT TEAR

**Description:** The anterior cruciate ligament (ACL) is the most commonly injured ligament in the knee. Tearing of the ACL can be classified as complete or partial. Other associated injuries such as O'Donoghue's unhappy triad includes, in addition to the tearing of the ACL, tearing of the posterior horn of the medial meniscus and partial tearing of the medial collateral ligament.

**Etiology:** Injury to the ACL can occur if the knee is (1) externally rotated and abducted with hyperextension, resulting in direct forward displacement of the tibia, or (2) internally rotated with the knee in full extension.

**Epidemiology:** Injury to the ACL tends to be highly associated with athletic sports (e.g., soccer and basketball) and seems to occur more commonly in females than males.

**Signs and Symptoms:** Patients usually present with pain and loss of function of the knee.

**Imaging Characteristics:** MRI is the recommended modality for evaluating the ACL with an accuracy rate of 95 to 100 percent for complete tears. To better visualize the ACL, the knee should be externally rotated 15 to 20 degrees to align the ligament in the sagittal plane.

### MRI
- The normal anterior cruciate ligament is seen as a band of low signal intensity.
- T2-weighted sagittal images are recommended for the evaluation of the ACL.
- Disruption of the ACL with no normal appearing fibers identified.
- Accuracy of MRI for the ACL is extremely high (95 to 100 percent).
- There may be associated findings such as joint effusion, meniscal tear, collateral ligament tear, or bone bruise.

**Treatment:** Complete tearing of the ACL is usually treated surgically. Partial tears are treated symptomatically.

**Prognosis:** Depends on the severity of the injury and other related injuries to the knee.

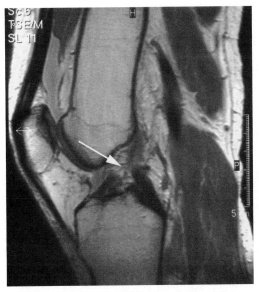

**FIGURE 1. Complete Tear of the Anterior Cruciate Ligament.** T1-weighted sagittal image through the intercondylar notch demonstrates the ACL to be disrupted (*arrow*).

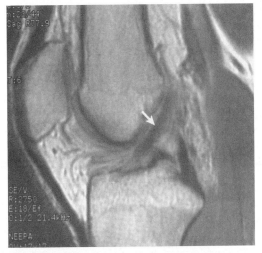

**FIGURE 2. Normal Anterior Cruciate Ligament.** T1-weighted image of normal anterior cruciate ligament (*arrow*).

# BAKER CYST

**Description:** A Baker cyst, also known as popliteal cyst, is a distended bursa located in the semimembranous/semitendinous bursa of the popliteal region of the knee.

**Etiology:** A Baker cyst can be produced by either a herniation of the synovial membrane or leakage of synovial fluid.

**Epidemiology:** These cysts may result from meniscal injuries, articular cartilage damage, collateral and cruciate ligament injuries, rheumatoid arthritis, loose bodies, and internal derangement of the knee.

**Signs and Symptoms:** Baker cysts may go unnoticed; however, when they are symptomatic, they manifest with edema and swelling.

### Imaging Characteristics:

### MRI
- T1-weighted images reveal a hypointense cyst.
- T2-weighted images demonstrate a hyperintense cyst.
- May show associated meniscal tears and joint effusion.

**Treatment:** May require resection if symptoms persist.

**Prognosis:** Good.

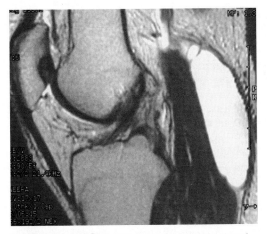

**FIGURE 1.  Baker Cyst.** T2-weighted sagittal (A) and axial (B) MR of the knee demonstrate a large oval high signal mass in the posterior medial aspect of the medial head of the gastrocnemius muscle consistent with a Baker cyst.

# BONE CONTUSION (BRUISE)

**Description:**   Bone contusions, also known as bone bruises or microtrabecular fractures are injuries to the trabecular that occur as a result of an impaction force.

**Etiology:**   Injury to the bony trabeculae usually results from an impaction force.

**Epidemiology:**   Most commonly involves the tibial plateau or the femoral condyles. There is a high incidence of bone bruises in patients with tears to their anterior cruciate ligament.

**Signs and Symptoms:** Patient presents with pain and a history of an injury.

**Imaging Characteristics:**   Radiographs are usually normal. MRI is very sensitive in detecting bony injuries.

## MRI
- T1-weighted images show low signal intensity within the bony area affected.
- Hyperintense signal intensity is seen in the bony area affected on T2-weighted images.
- STIR images show high signal intensity at the area of injury.
- The location of the bony injury may indicate associated soft-tissue injuries.
- Good for evaluation of associated ligament and meniscal injury.
- Useful for follow-up evaluation, especially in children.

**Treatment:**   Conservative treatment with a delay in returning to normal activity.

**Prognosis:**   Most bone contusions resolve without complications.

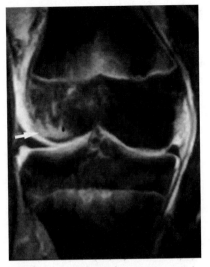

**FIGURE 1. Bone Contusion.** STIR coronal MRI shows focal increased signal intensity (*arrow*) of the medial femoral condyle.

# MENISCAL TEAR

**Description:**  A meniscal tear is an injury resulting in a tearing of the crescent-shaped fibrocartilage (meniscus) of the knee joint.

**Etiology:**  Tearing of the menisci may result from acute trauma, repetitive trauma, and progressive degeneration.

**Epidemiology:**  Meniscal tears usually occur as a result of athletic-related injuries. Nonathletic injuries, however, can occur in the aging population. Medial meniscal tears are more common than lateral meniscal tears. Meniscal tears can be associated with anterior cruciate ligament and medial collateral ligament tears, also known as the terrible triad or O'Donoghue sign.

**Signs and Symptoms:**  Pain and discomfort in mobility accompany meniscal tears.

## Imaging Characteristics:

### MRI
- T1-weighted or proton density weighted images are the most sensitive for diagnosis of meniscal tear.
- Normal meniscus appears as a low signal.
- Meniscal tear appears as a high signal.
- Meniscal tears may be longitudinal (traumatic) or horizontal (degenerative).
- Meniscal tear may be associated with an anterior cruciate ligament tear, medial collateral ligament tear, joint effusion or Baker cyst.

**Treatment:**  Depending on the extent of the injury, treatment may vary from physical therapy to meniscectomy.

**Prognosis:**  Varies depending on the extent of injury and other related factors such as age. The patient is encouraged to make a gradual recovery.

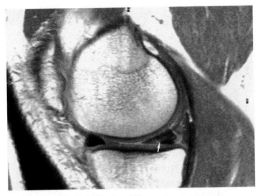

**FIGURE 1. Medial Meniscal Tear.** Proton density sagittal image of the knee demonstrates a horizontal tear (*arrow*) of the posterior horn of the medial meniscus that extends to the undersurface.

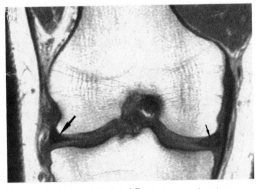

**FIGURE 2. Medial Meniscal Tear.** Proton density coronal image of the knee shows a complex tear (*thin arrow*) of the posterior horn of the medial meniscus compared with a normal (*thick arrow*) homogenous low-signal intensity of the lateral meniscus.

# Osteosarcoma

**Description:** An osteosarcoma is the most malignant primary bone tumor.

**Etiology:** In general, there is no known cause. However, radiation is a predisposing factor associated with the development of bone cancer. Genetic involvement is linked to patients with retinoblastoma.

**Epidemiology:** Primary bone cancers are rare, affecting approximately 1 in 100,000 persons. Approximately 4000 to 5000 cases are reported annually. These bone tumors are commonly located in the area of the knee, distal femur, or the proximal tibia. This cancer is generally seen in the younger population, ranging from the early teens to early twenties. Males are more commonly affected than females.

**Signs and Symptoms:** Patients present with pain, maybe a lump, or both. Approximately 10 percent of the patients who seek medical attention have already developed metastasis at the time of their initial evaluation. There is a great tendency for osteosarcomas to metastasize to the lungs.

**Imaging Characteristics:** Plain x-rays are very useful and should be done first. CT is good for the evaluation of bone. MRI is excellent for soft-tissue evaluation.

## CT
- Demonstrates bony destruction of the affected area.

## MRI
- T1-weighted images shows tumor as low signal intensity.
- T2-weighted images appear as high signal intensity.
- Disruption of the cortex.
- Associated soft-tissue mass.
- MR is the imaging modality of choice for the evaluation of the extent of the tumor.

**Treatment:** Surgical resection followed with chemotherapy.

**Prognosis:** Depends on the staging, if the cancer has spread to other parts of the body (i.e., lung or bone).

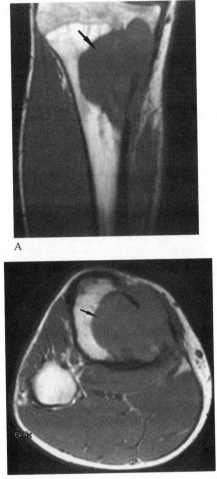

A

B

**FIGURE 1. Osteosarcoma.** T1-weighted
coronal (A) and axial (B) MRI show large
low signal intensity (*arrow*) mass involving
the medial aspect of the proximal tibia. There
is disruption of the cortex with extension of
the tumor medially.

# Posterior Cruciate Ligament Tear

**Description:** The posterior cruciate ligament (PCL) may appear with injuries categorized as consisting of ligamentous edema or hemorrhage, partial tearing, or complete tearing of the ligament.

**Etiology:** Tearing of the posterior cruciate ligament occurs as the result of a posterior force directed to the flexed knee or forced hyperextension.

**Epidemiology:** Tearing of the PCL occurs frequently in patients diagnosed with dislocation of the knee. Posterior cruciate ligament tears are not as common as anterior cruciate ligament tears.

**Signs and Symptoms:** Injuries to the knee involving tearing of the posterior cruciate ligament present with pain, loss of motion or disability, and the possibility of vascular and neurological complications.

## Imaging Characteristics:

### MRI
- T1- and T2- weighted images demonstrate the normal PCL as a low signal structure.
- T1-weighted images show poorly defined PCL.
- In acute tears, fluid and edema appear bright (hyperintense) with a high signal on T2-weighted pulse sequences.

**Treatment:** Depending on the severity of the injury, surgical intervention may be performed when there has been a tearing of the posterior cruciate ligament.

**Prognosis:** Depending on the degree of injury and other factors such as method of treatment and the patient's history, the patient's recovery and outcome may vary.

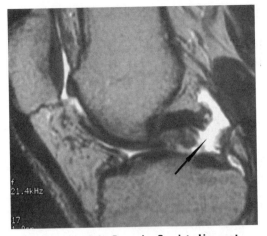

**FIGURE 1. Tear of the Posterior Cruciate Ligament.**
T2-weighted sagittal image of the knee demonstrate
a defect in the posterior cruciate ligament. There is
high signal intensity fluid collection at the site of the
tear (*arrow*).

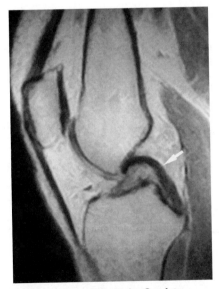

**FIGURE 2. Normal Posterior Cruciate
Ligament.** T1-weighted image of a normal
posterior cruciate ligament (*arrow*).

# QUADRICEPS TEAR

**Description:** A tearing or rupturing of the tendon of the quadriceps muscle usually occurs transversely and at the osteotendinous junction.

**Etiology:** Usually occurs as a result of forced muscle contraction or trauma.

**Epidemiology:** These injuries occur in the young athlete with either forced muscle contraction or direct trauma, or in the elderly, through a degenerative area.

**Signs and Symptoms:** Patient presents with pain at the site of the injury.

**Imaging Characteristics:** MRI is the imaging modality of choice.

**MRI**
- MRI is helpful in determining if the tear is partial or complete.
- Disruption or discontinuity of the quadriceps tendon.
- Increased signal intensity of the muscle/tendon on T2-weighted images.

**Treatment:** Surgical repair is required as soon as possible.

**Prognosis:** In general, the results are good.

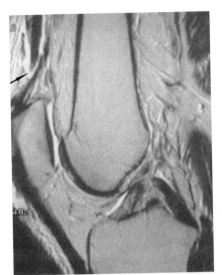

**FIGURE 1. Quadriceps Tear.**
T2-weighted sagittal
MR image shows disrup-
tion (*arrow*) with area of
increased signal intensity
in projection of the
quadriceps tendon.

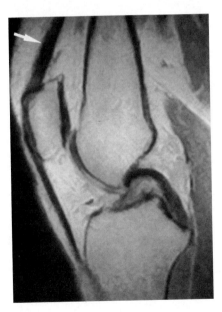

**FIGURE 2. Quadriceps.**
Normal quadriceps ten-
don (arrow).

# RADIOGRAPHIC OCCULT FRACTURE

**Description:** A fracture that is difficult to see radiographically, such as a stress fracture. These fractures are considered to be occult or equivocal fractures and may be evaluated with MRI. Historically, radionuclide bone scans were performed to evaluate these injuries; however, MRI has proven to be cost-effective, efficient, and able to detect these types of bony injuries.

**Etiology:** These fractures occur as a result of trauma or metabolic disorder.

**Epidemiology:** Occult fractures can occur at any age. Stress fractures in children and adults are associated with athletic activities; in the elderly, they can occur as a result of a metabolic disorder.

**Signs and Symptoms:** Patient presents with pain in the area of the injury.

## Imaging Characteristics:

### MRI
- T1-weighted images show the fracture as low-signal intensity.
- STIR images show the edema and hemorrhage associated with the fracture line as a high-signal intensity.

**Treatment:** Depends on the type and location of the fracture.

**Prognosis:** Generally good with early diagnosis and treatment. Avascular necrosis of the femoral head is a complication of the femur near the fracture.

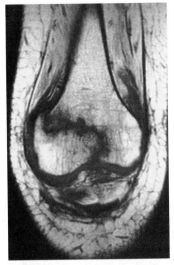

**FIGURE 1. Fracture of the Medial Femoral Condyle.** T1-weighted coronal MR image of the knee shows oblique fracture (low signal) of the medial femoral condyle extending to the articular margin or joint space. Note that the plain x-rays of the knee were negative.

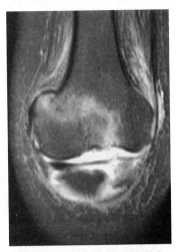

**FIGURE 2. Fracture of the Medial Femoral Condyle.** STIR coronal MR image of the knee (same patient as in Figure 1) shows an oblique fracture of the medial femoral condyle as high signal.

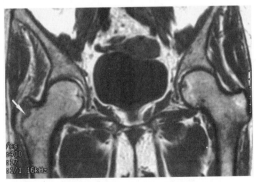

**FIGURE 3. Fracture of the Greater Trochanter.** T1-weighted coronal MRI of the pelvis shows a fracture of the greater trochanter of the right femur (*arrow*). Note that the plain x-rays of the hip were negative.

# UNICAMERAL (SIMPLE) BONE CYST

**Description:**  Unicameral bone cyst, sometimes referred to as simple bone cyst, are fluid-filled cysts. This bone cyst may present as a single-chambered cyst, or with a bubbly, multichambered appearance.

**Etiology:**  The cause of these benign lesions is unknown.

**Epidemiology:**  Unicameral bone cysts represent approximately 3 to 5 percent of the primary bone tumors. Although unicameral bone cysts typically present in the first two decades of life, approximately 80 percent of these cases commonly occur between the ages of 3 and 14 years. In approximately 90 percent of the cases, these bone cysts affect the proximal humerus, proximal femur, and proximal tibia. There is a male predominance of 3:1.

**Signs and Symptoms:**  This bony lesion is typically asymptomatic unless fractured. Approximately 67 percent of patients present with a pathologic fracture. Pain and loss of function accompany a fracture.

**Imaging Characteristics:**  Plain x-rays are usually diagnostic. MRI should always be correlated with plain films.

## CT
- The fluid-filled cyst appears hypodense.

## MRI
- This fluid-filled cyst is seen as a homogeneous low signal intensity on a T1-weighted image.
- T2-weighted images demonstrate high signal intensity.

**Treatment:**  Surgical intervention is the treatment of choice.

**Prognosis:**  Good; this is a benign tumor, with a small chance of recurrence.

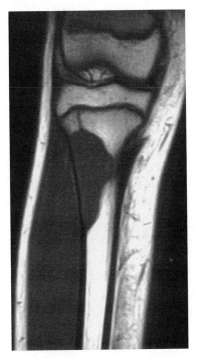

**FIGURE 1. Unicameral Bone Cyst.** T1-weighted coronal MRI shows low signal intensity lesion involving the proximal tibia.

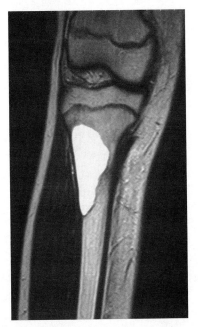

**FIGURE 2. Unicameral Bone Cyst.** T2-weighted MRI shows well-defined high signal intensity mass of the proximal tibia. The cortex is intact and there is no associated soft-tissue mass.

# ANKLE AND FEET

## ACHILLES TENDON TEAR

**Description:** The Achilles tendon, tendo calcaneus, is the longest and strongest tendon in the foot and ankle. Tearing of the Achilles tendon may be classified as either partial or complete.

**Etiology:** Tearing of the Achilles tendon usually results from indirect trauma such as athletic or strenuous activities.

**Epidemiology:** Athletic-related injuries can result at any age. Injuries associated with strenuous activities are most common between 30 and 50 years of age. Achilles tendon tears occur more commonly in males than females.

**Signs and Symptoms:** Patients usually present with pain, local swelling, and an inability to raise their toes on the affected side.

**Imaging Characteristics:** MRI is the useful modality for the detection of an Achilles tendon tear.

### MRI
- MRI is accurate in demonstrating partial and complete tears and following the progress of healing.
- Partial tear show increased signal intensity within the tendon on T2-weighted images.
- Complete tear shown as a wavy and lax tendon or discontinuity, retraction, and fraying of the ends. Increased signal at the site of the tear.
- T2-weighted double echo sagittal and axial images are the most useful.

**Treatment:** Partial tearing of the Achilles tendon may not require surgical intervention. Instead, immobilization and reduced weight bearing may be more appropriate. Patients with complete tears are candidates for surgical intervention.

**Prognosis:** The patient's outcome may vary depending on the extent of injury and method of treatment. Other factors to consider include the patient's age and mobility.

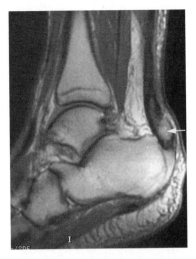

**FIGURE 1. Achilles Tendon Tear.**
T1-weighted sagittal MR of the
ankle demonstrates thickening
and intrasubstance increased
signal (*arrow*) within the distal
Achilles tendon, consistent with
a chronic tear.

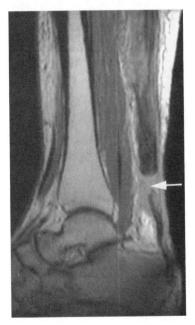

**FIGURE 2. Achilles Tendon Tear.**
T1-weighted sagittal MR of the
ankle demonstrates a complete
acute tear (*arrow*) of the Achilles
tendon near the musculotendi-
nous junction.

# BIBLIOGRAPHY

Berquist T H (ed): (*MRI of the musculoskeletal system*, 4th ed. Philadelphia: Lippincott Williams & Wilkins, 2001.

Canale S T (ed): *Campbell's operative orthopaedics*, 9th ed., vols. 1–4. St. Louis: Mosby-Year Book, 1998.

Cardenosa G: *Breast implant companion*. Philadelphia: Lippincott-Raven, 1997.

Castillo M: *Neuroradiology companion: Methods, guidelines and imaging fundamentals*. Philadelphia: JB Lippincott, 1995.

Cotran RS, Kumar V, Collins T eds: *Robbins pathologic basic of disease*, 6th ed. Philadelphia: W B Saunders, 1999.

Dambro MR (ed): *Griffith's 5-minute clinical consult*, 7th ed. Baltimore: Lippincott Williams & Wilkins, 1999.

Edelman RR, Hesselink JR, Zlatkin MB (eds): *Clinical magnetic resonance imaging*, 2nd ed., vols. 1 and 2. Philadelphia: WB Saunders, 1996.

Grossman RI, Yousem DM: *Neuroradiology:* The requisites. St. Louis: Mosby-Year Book, 1994.

Handbook of diseases. Springhouse, PA: Springhouse, 1996.

Harnsberger HR: *Handbook of head and neck imaging*, 2nd ed. St. Louis: Mosby, 1995.

Kriss VM: *Handbook of pediatric radiology*. St. Louis: Mosby, 1998.

Lee JKT, Sagel SS, Stanley RJ, Heiken JP (eds): *Computed body tomography with MRI correlation*, 3rd ed., vols. 1 and 2. Philadelphia: Lippincott-Raven Publishers, 1998.

Manaster BJ: *Handbook of skeletal radiology*, 2nd ed. St. Louis: Mosby-Year Book, 1997.

Moss AA, Gamsu G, Genant HK: *Computed tomography of the body: With magnetic resonance imaging*, vols. 1–3. Philadelphia: WB Saunders, 1992.

Murphy GP, Lawrence W Jr, Lenhard RE Jr (eds): *American cancer society textbook of clinical oncology*, 2nd ed. Atlanta: American Cancer Society, 1995.

Osborn AG, Tong KA: *Handbook of neuroradiology: Brain and skull*, 2nd ed. St. Louis: Mosby, 1996.

Rowland LP (ed): *Merritt's neurology*, 10th ed. Philadelphia: Lippincott Williams & Wilkins, 2000.

Sartoris DJ: *Musculoskeletal imaging: The requisites*. St. Louis: Mosby-Year Book, 1996.

Sider L (ed): *Introduction to diagnostic imaging*. New York: Churchill Livingstone, 1986.

Stark DD, Bradley WG Jr (eds): *Magnetic resonance imaging,* 3rd ed., vols. 1–3. St. Louis: Mosby, 1999.

Stern EJ (ed): *Trauma radiology companion: Methods, guidelines and imaging fundamentals.* Philadelphia: Lippincott-Raven, 1997.

Tierney LM, McPhee SJ, Papadakis MA (eds): *Current medical diagnosis and treatment,* 40th ed. New York: Lange Medical Books/McGraw-Hill, 2001.

Woodruff WW: *Fundamentals of neuroimaging.* Philadelphia: WB Saunders, 1993.

Yochum TR, Rowe LJ: *Essentials of skeletal radiology,* vols. 1 and 2. Baltimore: Williams & Wilkins, 1987.

# INDEX